100 STEPS
to a
LEAN
BODY

KATARINA NOLTE

For P.

"It is better to take many small steps in the right direction than to make a great leap forward only to stumble backward." ~*Old Chinese Proverb*
400 Motivational Weight Loss Quotes
http://www.fitnessforweightloss.com/helpful-weight-loss-quotes/

TABLE OF CONTENTS

DISCLAIMER

The statements and information in this book have not been evaluated by the FDA. It is not intended to treat, diagnose, cure, mitigate or prevent any disease. The content provided is for informational purposes only. Before starting any health or wellness program always seek the advice of your physician or other qualified, licensed health professional. Neither the author nor publisher take responsibility for any possible consequences from any treatment, procedure, exercise, dietary modification, action or application of medication which results from reading or following the information contained in this information. The publication of this information does not constitute the practice of medicine, and this information does not replace the advice of your physician or other health care provider.

Are you having trouble losing weight? Are you dealing with stubborn fat? Are you eating healthy and exercising and find yourself still unable to reach your optimal weight? Are you having problems finding clothing that fits you due to problem areas? Are you choosing clothing that hides your problem areas over the types of clothing you really like? Do you experience periodic bloating and embarrassing water retention? Are you tired of it all and absolutely serious about getting lean for good?

If any of the above applies to you, read "100 Steps to a Lean Body" and make it happen.

*I would like to express my gratitude to all the
people who publish and otherwise share practical
information on the subject of wellness.*

INTRODUCTION

Over one billion people are overweight and
nearly 600 million people worldwide are obese.
Annual obesity related expenses in the United
States are in the hundreds of billions of dollars.
The fattest people in the world can be found in
the United States where over 60% of adults are
overweight and over 30% are obese. Such
excesses in body fat have been associated with
hormonal imbalances, depression, sexual and
reproductive problems, cardiovascular disease,
diabetes, and cancer, and most of these
conditions are greatly influenced by a state
known as estrogen dominance. Estrogen
dominance is most likely to occur in individuals
whose bodies store too much internal (organ fat)
and/or external body fat (below the skin layer).
Body fat contains, both, endogenous estrogen
(produced by the body) and exogenous estrogen
(produced directly or indirectly by industrial
processes). The main focus of **"100 Steps to a
Lean Body"** is to remove wastes and toxins and
prevent future accumulation. These toxic wastes
include xenoestrogens in the form of industrially
processed food products, as well as other
sources like household and personal care
products.

You will learn what to eat and what to avoid or eliminate and what to do in order to increase your body's natural abilities to dispose of wastes and toxins. The information provided is short and to the point and is written in plain language that anyone can understand. If you follow the steps suggested in **"100 Steps to a Lean Body"** you will greatly improve your muscle to fat ratio and reduce or eliminate future weight problems. **"100 Steps to a Lean Body"** is written for people who are seriously interested in achieving these goals. If you selectively apply some of the steps suggested you will not achieve your optimal muscle to fat ratio. If you do apply all the steps suggested and invest time and patience into reaching your goals, you will succeed. In other words, this is not a get lean quick guide unless you have something like half a pound of excess fat which would be mostly water anyway. In such cases you can benefit from few of the suggestions you may not have tried in the past.

The group of people who most commonly experiences long term fat gain consists of individuals in the middle age range. At least half the people over the age of 30 begin to store so-called stubborn fat, the kind that often stays with you for the rest of your life. This is because this type of fat gain is the direct result of the typical lifestyle changes that occur around that age and thereafter. It is because around that age we simply stop moving and increasingly assume the position of mature individuals who no longer obsess over their figure. And, so, we pack on pounds. An average of 10-20 pounds each decade, to be precise. What this means is that one of the most obvious reasons for the world getting fatter is that the world is getting older. More and more people are living longer lives, lives which are often extended with a greater availability of processed foods and pharmaceuticals, as well as more opportunities to be a consumer. Of the physically lazy sort, of course.

Children and youths growing up today suffer the same misfortune by adapting to modern society's standards of spending their lives sitting on their behinds instead of following their natural instincts and being physically as active as possible. More and more people live in cities and suburbs with few natural, open spaces where young and old can safely gather and play sports, dance, swim, etc. Cities and suburbs alike are increasingly designed to serve vehicles, retail and industry over non-consuming pedestrians. Even shopping and other errands are increasingly done via the internet, phone or mail. Going to restaurants, events and movie theaters means sitting in a vehicle, sitting at the destination, sitting in a vehicle again and then sitting at home. Other than short walks from and to a vehicle and getting a quick lunch during lunch breaks, most people today spend their waking hours sitting or standing.

Obesity has been declared to be an ever growing pandemic against which no universal solutions exists as of yet. One of the main reasons for the various experts and authorities not being able to provide universal and concrete solutions is the world economy which depends on consumption regardless of the consequences for our species and the quality of life on Earth as a whole. The increasingly miserable state of human health and happiness stands in direct parallel with the state of health of the rest of the planet. What is obvious is that we can only be healthy if we are in balance, that is, if our total body chemistry is in balance. In order to achieve such a balance we must live and consume in proportion to our needs instead of ideas pertaining to modernization and monetary profits. Given the out of control growth in dietary consumption, sometime in the near future, our species may arrive at a point of maximum modernization and monetary profits but not enough in the form of edible plants and animals.

We already live in a time where a 10% obesity rate among women is considered to be low, despite the fact that a mere 50 years ago, a tiny

splash in the human evolutionary history, one
had to travel the entire world to find the few
obese individuals in existence back then. In the
short-lived TV show "Jamie Oliver's Food
Revolution" we could see that today's children
are unable to name common vegetables. Some
didn't even know that French fries came from
potatoes. What this means is that the women,
the mothers, grandmothers, aunts, etc. did not
take the time to teach children about the most
basic of foods, nor have they taken the time to
prepare meals by using real food ingredients. As
a result, children, youths, and young adults
suffer the consequences in the form of fat gain
and related health problems, including
developmental and reproductive issues. These
examples show us that human society is in a
state of cultural decline that is so grave that it
endangers the future survival of our species and
many other species on our magnificent planet.

Our planet is giving us everything we need to
thrive and we denature these wonderful gifts to a
point that they make us fat and sick. As you will
see, at a certain point in the short book that is
"100 Steps to a Lean Body" I give you
suggestions in areas which you may not readily
associate with weight problems. You will realize
that your mindset has everything to do with
your current weight issues and your future
success following the reading of **"100 Steps to a**

Lean Body". When we see obese and excessively overweight individuals (even when this is our reflection in the mirror) we must raise the question of what goes through the mind of the affected person. Does the person care about balance and feeling overall well? What is the degree of self-denial and what is it that is missing and is being replaced by an unhealthy lifestyle? Ultimately, we arrive at the realization that something must not be right in our collective culture if this issue continues to multiply, which is exactly what has been happening since, at least, the 1980's.

One of the weight gain culprits is emotional eating. People get upset and soothe their emotions with food. When people 100 or more years ago experienced this phenomenon they would pull a carrot out of the ground or grab a fruit off a tree. Regardless of how much they overate, they could not become obese. In addition to the fact that people back then consumed real, unprocessed, garden fresh, whole foods, they also tended to spend their lives doing some type of physical work. Today's culture has made it almost impossible for the average person to even have access to garden fresh food, while, at the same time, providing an ever growing number of convenience stores which sell mostly unhealthy, industrially processed snacks, as well as fast food

14

restaurants and other places that offer the same
substandard food that, basically, amounts to a
variety of edible factory products. One of the
reasons our emotions lead us to eat more than
we need in terms of food volume is that we feel
lousy and lacking when our diets do not deliver
the required amounts of nutrients. It is simply a
situation in which our emotions reflect the
struggles our bodies are going through due the
pathetic diet we feed them.

From there, we get to a point at which we find
ourselves no longer able to control our bodies'
cravings for nutrition, which we then, however,
attempt to satiate with more junk, because it is
industrially processed food that makes up a
large part of the economy. Individuals and
countries don't get rich selling whole, garden
fresh produce. They do get rich selling brand
name snack bars and sodas, and all the other
food stuffs with practically unlimited shelf lives.
The question that is not being asked is what
happens with that Frankenstein food after
consumption and whether it ever completely
leaves the body given that it contains few
nutrients, if any at all. The answers to such
questions get lost in the obesity statistics
mentioned above. For a period of time the
answer was to count calories and to discover the
best diet. This, as most people know by now, has
lead to the invention of one fad diet after

another, yo-yo dieting, starvation and bulimia, and health problems related to the constant changes in weight that so many people have suffered.

At this time there are multiple lifestyle diets which, if combined, would make for a perfect diet for the vast majority of people. These are: raw food diets (50-80% raw), the Paleolithic diet (or its closest copy), and the gluten-free diet. There are other diets that are quite effective but fall into the transitional diet category. These can be the elimination diet, done for the purpose of finding out which foods one exhibits an intolerance toward; and various short fasting or semi-fasting diets which serve to cleanse the body and sometimes prepare it for a drastic dietary change. Getting on such a preparatory diet or cleanse can be quite effective because once you introduce foods of a different type and/or quality, you may relatively quickly get used to the new lifestyle diet. Transitional diets and cleansing diets help remove problematic residues without which you no longer crave unhealthy or otherwise damaging foods. This, in turn, leads to the body being fitter and able to start burning fat sooner. At this point we must remember, once again, that **"100 Steps to a Lean Body"** is not a get lean quick diet.

While the main focus of **"100 Steps to a Lean Body"** is placed on switching from a diet based on industrially processed food to one that consists of real food, such a change alone does not produce the degree of success that the book is suggesting. In addition to dietary changes the steps include a series of supplements and many other details necessary to achieve optimal results. It is important that you take every detail contained in **"100 Steps to a Lean Body"** into account and incorporate it into your daily life. This is also one of the reasons why you will need time to achieve your personal optimum in terms of your muscle to fat ratio. **"100 Steps to a Lean Body"** is a holistic, all encompassing program meant for those who are ready to make all the changes necessary to change their figure for good. The typical modern environment we live in today, unfortunately, makes it difficult to be lean and remain lean indefinitely. Many individuals do begin to exercise regularly and even go as far as getting on any one of the comprehensive lifestyle diets that are available to us at present time, but they still struggle with their weight. For this reason, the focus of **"100 Steps to a Lean Body"** is, specifically, to lose fat and strengthen muscles in spite of the environmental obstacles. The combined steps will help you turn the fat burn and weight normalization switch on and keep it that way, but you must pay attention to detail and be

patient, thorough and focused for an extended
period of time until it becomes a habit. This is
what makes **"100 Steps to a Lean Body"** a
complete lifestyle changing program.

CHAPTER ONE: FOOD

1. STOP USING THE MICROWAVE

Microwaves not only destroy the nutritional value of food, but they also negatively influence the immediate environment in which they are located. To test this, get an EMF meter, measure the exposure by standing next to the microwave and then compare the measurement with that of a refrigerator, cell phone, or computer. Ideally remove the microwave and make sure not to consume microwaved food when eating out.

2. LEARN HOW TO COOK FROM SCRATCH

Cooking is very easy. All you need is a stove, a cast iron sautéing pan, a stainless steel cooking/steaming pot, and a glass baking dish. You can prepare any lunch or dinner by sautéing a piece of meat, poultry or fish for one or more minutes. Add some salad vegetables and a side of sautéed, steamed, baked or cooked vegetables. You can prepare a soup by combining a number of vegetables, grass-fed bone or bacon, and filtered water in a cooking pot and simmer them for 30-60 minutes. Desert can be a duo or trio of seasonal organic fruit, a fruit smoothie or a fruity, dairy and soy free protein shake. It's that simple.

3. STOP EATING INDUSTRIALLY PROCESSED FOOD

To be lean means having to loose fat and strengthen your muscles. In order for this to happen your system must be free of toxins, undigested food, and excess water weight. If you consume industrially processed food your digestion is impaired, you typically lack nutrients, and your body stores toxins and undigested food in fat cells and other tissues. This attracts pathogens which further impair your digestion and nutrient absorption. When your digestion is poor and you lack nutrients your body stores wastes instead of eliminating them. When your diet is low in nutrients and your body unable to absorb nutrients you cannot build muscles and other important tissues. In other words, your tissues lack density. This means that even if you are not overweight, you may look flabby. If you want your body and your skin to look taut, smooth and radiant, you need to dump the industrially processed food and go for high quality real food.

4. EAT REAL FOOD

What is real food? Real food is fresh organic food made from scratch that makes for the kind of meal where you know what's in it. No ingredient labels required. It is grass-fed meat and fat, wild caught fish, and organic produce like fresh salad vegetables and culinary herbs; organic

homemade soups containing cruciferous
vegetables, the onion family, tomatoes, and
grass-fed bacon or bone; organic, gluten free
spices; real, mineral-rich salt; etc. You get the
picture. One of the main reasons you must
switch to real food, aside from nutritional
density, is that by investing the time and energy
into the whole process of shopping for real food,
studying real food recipes, preparing real food,
and then enjoying the fruits of your loving labor,
you are working on the art of self love. By
switching from nutrient poor to nutrient rich
meals you are actively nurturing yourself and
your loved ones. And that's love. As for the
density: if you want strong, dense tissues, you
must consume nutrient dense food.

5. STOP EATING ARTIFICIAL SUGAR SUBSTITUTES

The problem with artificial sweeteners is that,
while they do sweeten foods and beverages, they
do not satisfy the so-called sweet tooth. This
means that the more sweeteners you use the
more sweet tasting foods and beverages you
crave. In other words, you achieve the exact
opposite of what you really want. If you want
that lean body to be the one you see in the
mirror, you must reduce your cravings for
sweets. To be successful with this endeavor, you
must find a way to achieve this without denying
yourself. Instead of denial, retrain your taste

buds and, as mentioned, your body doesn't get fooled by you feeding it pseudo sweets. So, again, go for the real thing.

6. EAT VERY SMALL AMOUNTS OF ORGANIC WHOLE CANE SUGAR AND RAW UNFILTERED HONEY

Which real food is naturally sweet? Plant foods are naturally sweet. There is fruit, of course. Some vegetables are on the sweet side. Then, there is honey. When shopping for honey make sure that it is pesticide-free and unfiltered. Unfiltered honey contains the honey itself, as well as the royal jelly and the bee pollen. If you purchase the superfood that is royal jelly, you will notice that it can be somewhat pricey. This means that the raw, unfiltered honey is not only extremely healthy in small amounts, but it also saves you money. Some types of honey are sold with the bees wax in it so as to sustain the authentic taste and aroma. And then there is sugar. The healthiest form of sugar is freshly pressed organic cane juice. If you don't live in a tropical paradise you can grow your own sugar cane plant. The plant can be grown outdoors as far north as the Southern U.S., Southern Europe, Pakistan, and Central China. The second healthiest is sucanat, which is whole sugarcane crushed into small pieces. There is also stevia (sweetleaf), but few people like it. Ideally, stick undenatured protein shakes made with homemade nut/seed milk and fresh or frozen fruit. This combination will provide you with enough sweetness and will prevent any potential cravings.

7. STOP EATING RAW CRUCIFEROUS VEGETABLES

Cruciferous vegetables like kale, collard greens, broccoli, cabbage, Brussels sprouts, and cauliflower are very healthy and useful for those looking to get lean. At the same time we hear that we should eat more raw food. Well, raw is great for weight loss and wellness, but not when it comes to the mentioned cruciferous vegetables. These must be cooked, steamed, sautéed, or fermented in order to become fully digestible. Secondly, we are told that fiber helps with slimming down because it supposedly stimulates elimination. Not true. At least not when it comes to indigestible (insoluble) fiber, also known as cellulose, as in wood, paper, cardboard, etc. You get the point. When these veggies are cooked, steamed, sautéed, or fermented, the important nutrients they contain are released and at the same time, these veggies are made easy for your system to process. In this state, you benefit from the nutrients and you eliminate better.

8. EAT LOTS OF RAW SALAD VEGETABLES

Prepare delicious salads every day and eat them twice a day. One large one and one or two small ones. Use a variety of lettuce including butter lettuce, arugula, radicchio, watercress, romaine, red leaf, green leaf, oak leaf, frisee, endive, mache, mizuna, and escarole lettuce; real mineral-rich salt, pepper, and other healthy spices; raw unfiltered fruit oils like olive, coconut, grapeseed or avocado oil; fresh, organic culinary herbs like parsley, cilantro, chives, dill, and mint; and other ingredients like onion, cucumber, tomato, olives, bell pepper, etc. Make sure to buy your produce in its original form (nothing precut) and if possible directly from the farm or garden. Salad produce is one of the few things we can get our hands on that are actually fresh. Remember: the more nutrient dense your diet is the closer you are to your goal. And you don't have to watch your salad oil consumption. Instead use it in generous amounts as long as it is raw and unfiltered. Make the salad the base of your meal. The rest can be any grass-fed meat or poultry or wild-caught fish. Again, you don't have to cut yourself short. Eat until you are full and feel free to eat every couple of hours from the time you wake up until 3 hours before bedtime. As long as you don't consume anything industrially processed, you can as much as you feel like.

9. STOP EATING CANNED VEGETABLES

The problem with canned foods is that they leach things like heavy metals (lead) and xenoestrogens (bisphenol A and phthalates) into the food. Not only do heavy metals exhibit estrogenic properties (metalloestrogens) and therefore fall into the category of the very problematic (and fattening) xenoestrogens, but the plasticizers used to line the cans are xenoestrogens as well. This means that if you are looking to gain fat and deal with water retention eat as many canned foods as your fat cells desire. Just joking. The point is that, once again, if you want leanness to be one of your attributes then steer clear of industrial toxins. As far as the nutritional quality of canned vegetables is concerned, fuggedaboutit. In addition to the above mentioned chemicals, they contain preservatives and who knows what else considering the manufacturers have no legal obligation to list all ingredients and processes applied to the food. Bottom line: if you want nutrients eat fresh food even if you end up cooking it. To see what I mean do the following: buy local veggies at the farmer's market and prepare a soup in the likes of a pot meal. Tons of veggies cut in bite size chunks, some filtered water, and grass-fed bacon chunks or bone. Simmer for 30-60 minutes. You will notice a delicious smell and an even better taste. Despite the fact that you killed some nutrients in the

cooking process, what you have is a delicious
and nutritious meal. Now try achieving the same
with canned veggies. Good luck. Lesson: use
your senses when determining the quality of a
whole food. The greater the variety of whole
foods you consume, the sharper your senses in
relation to real food will become.

10. EAT MORE COOKED, STEAMED, AND SAUTEED VEGETABLES

Vegetables, fruits, roots, and edible flowers like
spinach, kale, chard, cabbage, broccoli,
cauliflower, celery, artichoke, bell pepper, onion,
garlic, leeks, asparagus, turnip, eggplant,
squash, okra, parsley root, celeriac, kohlrabi,
carrot, arracacha, bamboo, cassava, daikon,
yam, ginger, horseradish, radish, Jerusalem
artichoke, jicama, mashua, parsnip, pignut,
jacón, and others can be cooked, steamed,
baked or sautéed together with raw, unfiltered
oils, and organic spices as side dishes. Aside
from an immense nutritional value, these types
of foods in their cooked form provide the much
needed satiation factor. When we change our
diet from the standard processed food to real
food with the goal of losing fat and strengthening
muscles for that lean look, hunger pangs and
cravings get in the way. When vegetables are
cooked and spiced tastefully, they satisfy the
cravings for starches and sugars. The latter is
also helped by the consumption of fresh fruits,

26

freshly pressed fruit juices, fruit smoothies, and fruit-protein shakes.

11. STOP EATING CANNED FISH & SEAFOOD

Here, again, we have the problems associated with cans and food that is not fresh. Secondly, there is the problem with fish and seafood and polluted seas and rivers, as well as the highly polluted fish farms. While I'd love to suggest you eat fish and seafood daily, due to pollution, overfishing, industrial style fishing and fish and seafood processing, such a recommendation is no longer valid. If it wasn't for pollution we would not only be very lean on a fish and seafood diet, but we would also thrive on many other levels. But, like said, no more.

12. EAT WILD CAUGHT FISH ONCE A WEEK

Wild caught seafood that is also unpolluted is hard to come by. Wild caught fish is available, at least according to the labels which may not always be fact based. Either way, fish is fantastic for a lean body, so do consume raw-marinated, sautéed, steamed or baked fish once a week. Fish oil capsules, fermented cod liver oil, sea vegetables (kelp), and microalgae (chlorella, spirulina, blue-green algae) can help you with your goal. The greens are good at helping the body detoxify heavy metals and other unwanted stuff. This, in turn, speeds up metabolism and helps you burn fat more effectively. Conclusion: a clean system is a lean system.

13. STOP EATING GLUTEN

Foods like grains, dairy, nuts, soy, peanuts, and eggs are known to cause problems like digestive issues, allergies and intolerances in many individuals. Most grains contain gluten, lectins, phytates, and other anti-nutrients which prevent proper digestion and nutrient absorption, and lead to nutritional deficiencies and weight gain in the form of fat gain and water retention. Even when the problematic grains are soaked and sprouted, they can cause similar issues. For this reason it is best to eliminate them and see what kinds of results their elimination brings. If you experience more energy, less water retention and a gradual satisfactory loss of fat, you may decide to steer clear of problematic grains or all grains indefinitely.

14. EAT SMALL AMOUNTS OF RAW CRACKERS AND OTHER RAW BREADSTUFFS

Raw crackers and raw breadstuff is typically made of mixtures of ground up, soaked and sometimes sprouted nuts and seeds, vegetables, culinary herbs, and spices. Most raw foodie foods are organic or wild. In other words, as free of toxins as possible. The ingredients are blended and dried in a dehydrator at temperatures of up to 118 degrees Fahrenheit so as to preserve things like enzymes, vitamins, and other delicate nutrients. If you have so far been unfamiliar with the raw foodie diet you will be astonished at its richness and creativity. Most people think that vegetarians, raw foodies, and vegans spend their days munching on carrot and celery sticks. Not so. Note: I do not recommend a diet free of meat, poultry and fish as they often produce nutritional deficiencies. If you, however, choose to take that route start by taking a year to consult nutritional specialists on the subject and read as much as you can on the specific subject of nutritional needs in terms of vitamins, minerals, amino acids, co-vitamins, enzymes, co-enzymes, and all the other good stuff.

15. STOP CONSUMING SOY/DERIVATIVES

The reason why soy makes you gain fat and retain water is that most soy and soy derivatives on the market are made from unfermented and often genetically modified soy. Even if the soy is organic, if it is unfermented it cannot be digested. If it cannot be digested you have to deal with issues like sluggish digestion, difficulties with nutrient absorption, nutritional deficiencies, constipation, excess estrogen (estrogen dominance), sluggish metabolism, lack of energy, water retention and fat gain. To avoid this you can consume tiny amounts of organic, fermented soy foods, but you must eliminate any

and all products containing unfermented soy
and soy derivatives. To avoid such products you
will have to discontinue the consumption of
more than half the foods at a typical
supermarket. Further, many such products'
ingredient lists do not specifically state 'contains
soy' or 'may contain soy' because food
manufacturers are under no legal obligation to
list every single ingredient or the traces thereof.
Due to the increase in allergies and intolerances,
however, many products do contain such
warnings.

16. EAT MORE RAW FERMENTED FOODS

When opting for fermented foods consider
making your own raw, lacto-fermented
vegetables at home. This way, you are in charge
of the ingredients, amounts, and the overall
quality of the preparation. Raw, lacto-fermented
foods are so-called living foods that contain
probiotics (friendly gut bacteria), thereby
supporting the entire process of digestion and
providing important nutrients. As noted,
thorough digestion, nutrient absorption and
nutrient density are integral to a lean body.
Examples of fermented foods include
sauerkraut, sauerkraut juice, kimchi, yogurt,
vegan coconut yogurt, etc. You can ferment
pretty much any vegetable or vegetable
combination. Some cultures consume fermented
fish (rakfisk, bagoong, etc.), meat (jamón ibérico,

salami, etc.), fruit (apple cider vinegar, atchara, nata de coco, etc.), and tea (kombucha, Pu-erh tea, etc.). Technically, cacao beans are fermented as well by letting them sit under banana leafs for a period of time. This may be one of the reasons why cacao is beneficial as long as it is consumed without added sugars/sweeteners or with minimal amounts of added sugar and preferably together with protein so as to prevent a spike in blood sugar, fat gain, etc. When it comes to fermented foods, you will derive most benefit from the consumption of homemade, organic, raw-fermented vegetables.

17. STOP EATING LOW QUALITY ANIMAL PRODUCTS

Low quality animal products come from unhealthy animals due to inappropriate diets, living conditions, and mistreatment. Your goal must be to eat as healthy as possible, because that is the only way to get the maximum amount of nutrients and to prevent toxins from accumulating and leading to fat gain and water retention. Things like dairy and processed meat are particularly problematic and counterproductive to your goals.

18. EAT MULTIPLE SMALL PORTIONS OF HIGH QUALITY ANIMAL PRODUCTS

Protein is essential to fat loss and overall balance, including that of fluids. Many people

31

are either unable to digest protein due to the protein being of low quality or due to their diet including foods that prevent protein digestion and absorption. If you suspect this to be one of your issues that lead to problems with weight and fat-to-muscle ratio, you will want to increase your consumption of protein powders like whey and hemp protein. Firstly, this will make it easier for your body to digest and absorb protein. Secondly, protein deficiency caused by the mentioned issues typically leads to cravings for sugars and starches. In other words, when your body is lacking protein, you are more likely to reach for processed junk food. Ideally consume 3 or 4 protein shakes daily. Make sure that your protein shakes are homemade; your protein pure, meaning unflavored, unsweetened, and undenatured (not heated past a certain temperature; that the liquid you use is hemp milk, filtered water, fresh coconut water, freshly pressed juice, or homemade presoaked nut/seed milk, and that your other ingredients, which may include things like fresh or frozen fruit, cacao powder, maca powder, beneficial herbs and supplements in powder form, ground nuts and seeds (presoaked), etc., are raw, organic and generally high in quality and freshness. The rest of your protein intake can consist of grass-fed meat and poultry and wild-caught fish. You will want 3-6 portions of no more than 20 grams of

protein each. This will help with satiation,
nutrition, energy, strengthening, and fat burn.

19. STOP CONSUMING DAIRY

When it comes to digestive problems, fat gain,
bloating, and water retention, dairy is often one
of the culprits. Some people switch from
conventional dairy to organic dairy to no avail.
Even raw organic dairy, which is the purest and
therefore easiest for the body to process, can
cause the above mentioned issues. To see if
dairy affects you negatively, try the elimination
diet for a few days or a few weeks. Eliminate all
dairy and see how you feel, overall. If you feel
better and notice less bloating, gas, and water
retention, look for dairy alternatives like
homemade dairy made out of fresh ripe or young
coconuts, homemade nut and seed dairy, and
store-bought hemp milk. Hemp milk is made
from hemp plant seeds which must be soaked,
and it is this soaking and the nature of the plant
that make it a less problematic dairy substitute.
See if you can find unsweetened hemp milk or
hemp seeds for homemade hemp seed dairy.
While raw, organic, homemade, unsweetened
and unflavored yogurt or kefir usually doesn't
cause any problems, cow milk dairy has recently
been found to be high in radiation.

20. CONSUME FRUIT (COCONUT) AND SEED (HEMP) DAIRY

For much of our existence, we have subsisted mostly on fruit. This is why fruit-based dairy and fruit-based culinary oils are so healthy. More often than not, foods that are healthy are least likely to cause fat gain and water retention. Coconut is antiviral, antibacterial, antifungal, anti-inflammatory, antiparasitic, and helps balance blood sugar, hormone and cholesterol levels, improves energy levels and digestion, and supports nutrient absorption. When used in cooking, coconut oil remains stable unlike other culinary oils. While unfiltered olive oil is best for cold meals like salads, unfiltered coconut oil is best for cooking and baking. Learn to make your own coconut milk, yogurt, and oil; flaxseed milk, and hemp milk. As already mentioned, the more you learn to prepare your own foods and beverages, the more control you have over the quality of your consumption and, ultimately, over your weight. Hemp seeds are anti-inflammatory and indirectly help balance hormones and cholesterol levels. When preparing nut or seed milk you must soak them first in order to reduce the amounts of naturally occurring antinutrients. Chestnuts contain the least phytic acid and are seasonal and therefore unavailable most of time. For these reasons chestnuts do not require soaking, which means that if they are available you can prepare chestnut milk within minutes. On the subject of homemade dairy alternatives: try consuming them without any ingredients meant to sweeten their taste. Then, add the absolute minimum amount of honey, cane juice, agave, fresh grapes or dates. The goal here is to learn to enjoy just a whiff of sweetness and be fully satisfied with it. This may take some time but it's worth it.

21. STOP EATING ROASTED NUTS AND SEEDS

Like grains and legumes (beans, lentils, peas, peanut), nuts and seeds contain antinutrients which disable the body from digesting protein. Protein is the most important base nutrient (along with water and carbohydrates). Our bodies are made of it. When we are unable to digest protein we become protein deficient and experience an array of imbalances. We often develop cravings for junk food, the habit of overeating, and resultant fat gain and water retention. Soaking grains, legumes, nuts and seeds helps a little in our ability to digest these foods (almost) completely. Roasted nuts and seeds are not soaked prior to being roasted and are therefore not conductive to your goal.

22. EAT SMALL AMOUNTS OF SOAKED NUTS AND SEEDS

Soaking nuts and seeds and using them to make homemade nut and seed milk and yogurt greatly improves their nutritional value because soaking and raw fermentation predigest the food and increase the availability of the nutrients contained within. If you rotate your use of coconut and nut/seed dairy substitutes, you end up consuming an overall moderate amount of nuts and seeds.

23. STOP CONSUMING LOW QUALITY SPICES

Many conventional spices and especially spice mixes contain additives which are not healthy and can cause problems with digestion and weight.

24. START CONSUMING HIGH QUALITY SPICES

Opt for organic and pesticide-free spices and discover new spices so as to make your meals unique and add minute amounts of nutrients. Spices like cinnamon, maca, turmeric, curry, black pepper, cayenne pepper, crushed chili, garam masala, ginger, cumin, coriander, garlic, mint, parsley, oregano, and others are beneficial for weight loss. Avoid or eliminate condiments, dressings and conventional salt. Learn to prepare your own homemade sauces, dips, dressings, and marinades. Experiment. Have fun.

25. MACA

Maca helps balance hormones, normalize appetite and satiation, lift the mood, increase energy levels, burn fat, build muscles, and is overall health supportive. Maca is a root vegetable, so it, technically, can be consumed daily, but being a potent food, it might be more effective in rotation (on/off cycle). Maca is a superfood and should be raw and organic. When shopping for maca you will notice that bulk purchases of 16 ounce bags (or larger) are very inexpensive when compared to capsules. Raw, organic maca powder is also more practical, allowing you to use it as a food ingredient as well as a supplement. You can stir it into sauces, smoothies, protein shakes, and homemade, raw spreads, cookies, crackers, etc. It's a wonderful, tasty spice and it blends well with, both, sweet and salty foods.

26. SEA VEGETABLES

Seaweeds help cleanse the system of wastes and toxins. They deliver nutrients like chlorophyll, minerals and trace elements, and even some protein. Eat them like chips, sprinkle them on your food, stir them into your salads, and add them to your soups and sauces.

27. KELP, SPIRULINA, CHLORELLA

Supermodels are famous for consuming green foods. Green foods cleanse the system and help keep you slender.

28. SUPERFOODS

Superfoods like goji berries, maca, unfiltered raw honey, hemp and chia seeds, cacao, seaweeds (chlorella, kelp, spirulina, kombu, etc.), culinary herbs; raw, unfiltered oils like coconut and olive, and countless fruits and vegetables nourish your system and help rebalance it. When you rid yourself of excess fat and water, what you are really doing is creating a state of internal harmony.

29. GREEN AND RED POWDERS

Companies like Live Juice Powders, Garden of Life, Amazing Grass, Greens Plus, Powder Pure, and others produce and sell dried fruit and vegetable powders. Such powders are useful when there is no opportunity to drink freshly pressed fruit or vegetable juices. As mentioned, today's plants are not what they used to be in terms of nutrient density and drinking freshly pressed fruit or vegetable juices and fruit and vegetable powders, along with a real food diet, considerably raises the total amount of nutrients consumed. Nutrition is key for getting and keeping a strong, lean body.

30. COLORFUL

Grow your knowledge of food and make sure that you eat something different every week and every season. Learn about the countless types of fresh produce, fresh meats, fish, seafood, and culinary herbs and spices. Mix and match and experiment. Create your own recipes and discover your new favorites. Make your meals look good and take your time when eating.

31. STOP EATING 3 HOURS BEFORE BEDTIME

The body digests food for up to 4 hours. Going to sleep with a full stomach causes undigested food to sit in the gut until the next day because, once asleep, your digestion stops or slows down considerably. Going to bed with a full stomach can also lead to nightmares which you may or may not remember, but, which affect your mood the next day nonetheless. Firstly, you will want your food to be digested swiftly and completely. Secondly, you will want to be in a good mood so as to be better able to adapt to your new diet and lifestyle and ultimately achieve your goal of having a lean body. If you eat real food, drink your protein shakes, smoothies and freshly pressed fruit and vegetable juices, take quality supplements, exercise, and manage your stress with healthful, pleasant methods, you will not be hungry at bedtime. You will feel the need for sleep and not for food. So eat all day and then stop 3 hours before bedtime.

CHAPTER TWO: NUTRITIONAL SUPPLEMENTS

32. STOP WASTING YOUR MONEY ON GET LEAN QUICK MAGIC POTIONS

Get lean quick supplements consist of combinations of ingredients which may work for some people for a period of time or not at all. Firstly, without switching from industrially processed food to real food and regular aerobic and anaerobic exercise, you are, at best, losing water only to regain it later. Such combo supplements are typically overpriced as well. If they contain herbs, the effect dwindles with time because herbs must be rotated (cycled) in order to work in the long run.

33. BUY PURE SUPPLEMENTS AND HERBS THAT WORK SLOWLY

Pure supplements are individually packaged vitamins, herbs, amino acids, etc. If, for example you consume a specific combination of amino acids they together will have one specific effect. If you take amino acids individually, you will get all the benefits of a given amino acid. If you take all the major amino acids together, they will compete with one another for absorption. This means that if you buy individual amino acids, you are able to take any one alone or combine

41

certain amino acids in order to achieve specific
results for a period of time. To avoid confusion:
protein powder is a whole protein food. Protein
or any sort, be it vegetable or animal-based,
consists of amino acids, but in order for the
body to absorb these amino acids, it must break
down the protein. For this reason, protein
powders designed for athletes, for example, are
predigested for better absorption of amino acids.
This, however, doesn't mean that your body will
be able to absorb each amino acid found in a
given protein powder because the amino acids
compete with one another. Secondly, each
individual is unique and how and to what extent
your system will benefit from a nutrient varies.
This is another reason why it is best to research
nutrients, nutritional supplements, herbs, etc.,
purchase them individually packaged, and
experiment by consuming different
combinations, followed by rotation (on/off cycle).
Herbs and nutritional spices can be purchased
inexpensively in bulk and free of pesticides, etc.,
at Mountain Rose Herbs. In the case of herbs,
follow the same process: do your research, learn
how to use herbs, and see what works for you,
followed by rotation (cycling) for best results.

34. STOP BELIEVING THAT A LITTLE EXTRA PROTEIN WILL BE ENOUGH

While we all have individually unique nutritional
requirements, protein is the most essential

nutrient for humans. Without it growth, development and regeneration are impossible. Most importantly, fat burn and an increase in muscle strength cannot happen without a sufficient amount of daily protein intake. Note that a minimum daily requirement is not the same as the amount which is adequate for a person who is on a program focused on fat burn, muscle strengthening and weight loss.

35. UNDERSTAND HOW PROTEIN GETS USED UP

Consume no more than 20 grams of protein at any one time. Consume 20 grams of protein every couple of hours. With daily exercise, consume your protein 5 times per day. Example: one small hamburger patty and two chicken breasts make a combined 60 grams of protein. These could be 3 meals if you include soup, side, and/or salad. Add to that 2 protein shakes, each containing 20 grams of protein. Total for the day: 100 grams of protein divided into 3 meals and 2 snacks. You will also derive small amounts of protein from the plant foods you consume. For the average person who exercises every day and lives on real food, 120 grams of total protein consumed in a day would be ideal.

36. STOP CONSUMING FLAVORED AND SWEETENED PROTEIN POWDERS

Flavored and sweetened protein powders are often denatured. This means that they are processed at temperatures which change the protein structure making it difficult for the body to digest and derive nutrients (amino acids) from. Most foods heated at temperatures beyond the maximum temperatures created by sunlight (118 degrees Fahrenheit) tend to destroy nutrients like vitamins, enzymes, co-vitamins, co-enzymes, amino acids, etc. Denaturing drastically lowers the quality of a given food and, as mentioned, your goal must be to derive as much nutrition as possible from the foods and beverages you consume.

37. CONSUME PURE UNDENATURED PROTEIN POWDER

Pure undenatured protein powder tastes best, thereby, helping you fine-tune your taste buds and adjust your needs for sweetness down to the level found in nature (fresh fruit, honey). Most industrially processed foods and sweetened protein powders are excessively sweetened. You will notice this in time. Pure undenatured protein powder allows you to prepare you protein drinks with a single protein powder and experiment with whatever flavors you like on a given day. You can add any type of fruit, vegetable, and spice you feel like as long as it is

44

fresh, organic, and/or wild. Once again, you control what goes into your system.

38. STOP CONSUMING ANTIBIOTICS

Antibiotics kill friendly bacteria in the gut. This leads to the body being unable to digest food properly and draw nutrients out of the food consumed. It also causes constipation which I covered in my book "So Long Constipation, Part 1". This, in turn, leads to bloating, gas, fat gain, and water retention.

39. CONSUME PROBIOTICS

Probiotics and prebiotics are found in fermented foods and raw foods. Garden fresh, raw foods, in particular, are rich in prebiotics which turn into probiotics (friendly gut bacteria) during digestion. Probiotics support digestion, absorption, and elimination. They help balance hormones and weight.

40. L-CARNITINE

Carnitine is an amino acid found in protein-rich foods including meat, poultry, game, etc. Carnitine helps the body burn fat sooner. Normally, the body burns any available carbs first, but with more carnitine, or simply more grass-fed meat, the body is more likely to use fat for energy. As mentioned, by consuming the amount of protein (amino acids, once broken down) your body needs, you burn more fat and gain more strength which, together, results in the lean look you want.

41. CHROMIUM PICOLINATE

Chromium is a mineral trace element found in supplemental form as well as in meat, fish, seafood, eggs, greens, bulbous and root vegetables. Chromium helps balance blood sugar and pressure. Balanced blood sugar levels make it easier to properly digest food and eliminate wastes, burn fat, and lose excess weight.

42. L-GLUTAMINE

Glutamine positively affects digestion, cleansing, fat burn, strength, and post-workout recovery. It is found in supplemental form and in protein-rich foods including meat, fish, poultry, eggs, and greens.

43. L-ARGININE/L-ORNITHINE

Arginine is an amino acid found in protein-rich foods like meat, fish, eggs, and green vegetables like dark leafy greens, parsley, coriander (cilantro), seaweeds, etc. Arginine helps burn fat and strengthen muscles. One of the reasons is that it, by itself, as well as in combination with orthithine, tyrosine, and lysine, helps produce the human growth hormone (HGH). Arginine works best in combination with ornithine. Arginine/ornithine combo supplements are

46

available in most places where nutritional
supplements are sold.

44. TYROSINE

Tyrosine is an amino acid found in protein-rich
foods, including meat, poultry, fish, seafood, and
greens (especially seaweeds). Tyrosine is
beneficial for an overall sense of balance. It can
help curb cravings for junk food, balance
hormones, (indirectly) burn fat, and improve
workout results.

45. LIQUID IONIC MINERALS

Most people today are deficient in minerals and
trace elements due to pollution and over-
farming. Supplement with liquid ionic minerals
and trace elements for optimal absorption. You
will have an easier time losing excess fat and
water.

46. VITAMIN D

Vitamin D is actually a hormone which we
normally get from sun exposure. Vitamin D
helps balance hormones, strengthens immunity,
lifts your mood, and helps you burn fat faster.
Vitamin D is available in supplemental form as
vitamins D3. By the way, the vitamin D2 added
to processed milk and store bought non-dairy
milk is useless. Vitamin D rich foods include fish
and seafood, meat, animal fat, and organ meat.

47. MULTIVITAMIN WITHOUT IRON

Make sure that your multivitamin does not
contain iron as iron prevents the absorption of
certain vitamins. Also, see that the percentages
shown on the label exceed 100% of the daily
recommended amounts. The daily recommended
amounts of nutrients are the absolute minimum
needed for survival. For optimal function,
considerably higher levels of nutrients are
needed. And, finally, we absorb only 50% or less
of the nutrients contained in supplements. You
may improve absorption somewhat by
consuming your multivitamins with food and
supplemental digestive enzymes.

48. VITAMIN C

Vitamin C is an essential vitamin we must
consume via food and supplements. Many fresh
fruits and vegetables, as well as meat, contain
vitamin C. When purchasing vitamin C
supplements, opt for those which include
bioflavonoids. You can take individual vitamin C
or C ester capsules throughout the day to
support cleansing and digestion.

49. VITAMIN B COMPLEX

Very many people are deficient in B vitamins. B
vitamins will help you relax and stay grounded
in your intention to get a lean body. They will
help you keep an optimistic outlook and bring
you closer to your goal. Fresh fruit and

vegetables, as well as meat and poultry contain B vitamins. They are also available in supplement form.

50. DIGESTIVE ENZYMES

Digestive enzymes are essential for two things: digestion and elimination. Very many people today suffer from digestive issues. One of the most common is a compromised ability to digest protein. If you are looking to cleanse the body of wastes and toxins you must not be deficient in amino acids which make up protein. Digestive enzymes also improve digestion by supporting nutrient absorption and waste elimination. Secondly, digestive enzymes, when taken away from food, help remove any surplus debris, metabolic wastes, and toxins out of the body. One of the reasons why people on an overwhelmingly raw diet lose their problem zones (stubborn fat), cellulite, and other annoyances is because the digestive enzymes naturally found in raw food have not been damaged by the heating of the food. So, if on top of that you take supplemental digestive enzymes, guess what happens? The surpluses of fat and water gradually dissolve.

51. GINSENG

Ginseng is an adaptogenic herb. Adaptogens help balance internal systems, including hormones. An improved hormonal balance leads to an improved muscle to fat ratio and less water retention.

52. CLA

Conjugated linoleic acid is found primarily in grass-fed and wild game ruminants and to a lesser extent in industrially grown meat, poultry and pork, as well as in animal milk and fat. CLA is also available in supplement form. It helps burn fat and less fat means stronger muscles. Fat depots contain estrogenic substances which prevent muscle building and maintenance. The less fat you carry the easier it is to stay lean. Note that the meat and fat from healthy animals will not make you fat as long as it is fresh. Cold cuts can be consumed on rare occasion, but are not advisable while on a fat loss program.

53. STOP YOUR DISBELIEF IN NUTRITIONAL SUPPLEMENTS

Today's soils are depleted of vital nutrients due to industrial farming and pollution. The plants we and our farm animals consume are, therefore, nutrient poor. This applies even to organic foods, even though organic foods often contain up to twenty times the nutrients when compared to conventional foods. Nutritional supplements can help you add the nutrients your food is lacking, at least to some extent. Many supplements are food based. These include herbs, roots, grasses, freeze dried fruit

and vegetable powders, sea vegetables (incl.
micro algae), protein powders, whole meal
powders, minerals and trace elements, fish oil,
vegetable based vitamins and provitamins, etc.
For best results, read "Prescription for
Nutritional Healing" by Phyllis A. Balch.

54. READ "PRESCRIPTION FOR NUTRITIONAL HEALING"

This book has been around forever and is
periodically updated and republished. It explains
what nutrients are and what they do. It consists
of different sections, including a section that
provides a full diet and supplement plan for
pretty much any common ailment.

CHAPTER THREE: CLEANSE

55. KEEP INFLAMMATION AT BAY

Inflammation is very common today, as is fat gain. This is because inflammation is a sign of stress. Mental stress, environmental stress, and the stress caused by ourselves. That is, us stressing about all the things that stress us out. The latter can be eliminated which is key to managing all of our combined stresses by taking charge and changing how we view stress. Secondly, we must put time aside for stress relieving activities. Note that you may hear how meat causes inflammation. What really causes inflammation, diet-wise, is industrially processed food and, more specifically, food based on and containing grains, corn and soy. Anti-inflammatory foods are most garden fresh fruits and vegetables, culinary herbs, fruit oils, and fish and seafood. Anti-inflammatory activities are time spent in nature, exercise, slow-deep breathing, swimming in natural bodies of water, and various relaxation methods including things like music and color therapy, massage, dancing, meditation, yoga, etc.

56. STOP THE TOXIC OVERLOAD

We live in a world full of toxic substances including those found in buildings, household

products, personal products, clothing,
electronics and vehicles. There is air pollution,
water pollution, soil pollution, toxic residue in
produce and animal products, you name it.
These toxins get stored in our bodies making us
fat, sluggish, and moody.

57. START ELIMINATING ANY POTENTIAL EXPOSURE TO TOXINS

Discover products that are free of toxins (or
almost free of them). Learn about simpler, more
natural ways for getting things done. Clean up
your diet and your household. Do internal
cleansing for your organs, consume more
greens, sweat often, and get an air cleaner and
some EMF protection for you home and
workplace.

58. STOP MESSING WITH YOUR DIGESTION

Industrially processed food and industrial
pollution of the environment wreak havoc on our
digestion. The body is overwhelmed, becomes
unable to rid itself of toxins and starts storing
fat and water.

59. READ "SO LONG CONSTIPATION, PART 1"

The most important venue of elimination is the
gut which is why we must pay close attention to
what we consume and how the foods and
beverages we consume make us feel. This is best
observed through the elimination diet which

53

helps us recognize which foods are most problematic and stop consuming them.

60. WOODEN MANUAL CELLULITE ROLLER

Rollers improve circulation, diminish tension, and can be useful to people affected by cellulite. If you have just begun exercising you may notice some muscle tension here and there. Do stretching exercises after each workout, use the rollers, get good sleep, and keep your muscles warm. You will notice that the more raw food you consume the better the tone and texture of your skin looks and feels like. After a year or so you may find that your problem areas are gone. Just like that. It is the difference between consuming industrially processed food and real food.

61. DRY BRUSHING

Dry brushing can be done a couple of times per week. It helps improve circulation, oxygenation, and the removal of internal wastes and toxins.

62. XENOESTROGEN CLEANSE

Xenoestrogens are estrogen-like substances derived from industrial products and processes. They include plastics and other synthetics, heavy metals (metalloestrogens), oral contraceptives and other estrogenic pharmaceuticals, cosmetics and personal care products, and household cleaners, detergents, deodorizers, etc. Metalloestrogens, in particular, are everywhere in our environment, air, water (including rain and natural bodies of water), soil, plants, animals, and human bodies. Easing this load is difficult but not impossible. Firstly, eat real food that is as fresh as possible. Secondly, exercise regularly. Thirdly, sweat regularly. Fourthly, spend as much time as possible in clean natural environments. Fifthly, explore and employ new relaxation methods.

63. HEAVY METAL DETOX

Detoxifying heavy metals clears the organs and tissues and improves overall functioning, circulation, metabolism, digestion, etc. As mentioned, the body holds an excess of fat and water as a means to set aside toxins which it cannot process at a given moment. Removing heavy metals reverses this process and you lose excess water and fat if you combine the detox with a real food diet and exercise. Green vegetables, green salads, sea vegetables, culinary herbs, and green vegetable powders can be of benefit. The same goes for herbs like milk thistle, cloves, garlic, and turmeric. Also, add liquid ionic minerals and trace elements, as well as magnesium, selenium, and zinc to your regimen.

64. HOT

Hot and spicy foods can help speed up metabolism and stimulate cleansing and elimination. Make sure that the food is fresh, organic and homemade and don't consume hot and spicy food if you don't enjoy it. Enjoyment of your lean body program is critical. The more pleasant and enjoyable you make it the closer you are to your goal.

65. STAY WARM

We all know that losing weight is easier during the summer months. Keeping your muscles warm helps you burn fat and maintain a high metabolic rate. It is also supportive when it comes to muscle conditioning, muscle recovery, and muscle building. By keeping warm all the time you are less likely to incur an injury or experience post workout muscle soreness.

66. START SWEATING REGULARLY

Sweating regularly is essential for the elimination of wastes and toxins. Upping the elimination of wastes and toxins helps reduce the amount of fat and excess water your body is holding, and makes strengthening your muscles and keeping your joints and tendons flexible easier. And, finally, sweating and keeping warm relaxes the body and the mind.

67. STOP THE NONSTOP ELECTROMAGNETIC POLLUTION

We are swimming in manmade energy fields. It has been estimated that we currently have something like a billion times more radiation in our environment than what is normally found in nature. Pollution equals stress. Just like we must eliminate, reduce and manage stress in order to be healthy and lean, we must eliminate, reduce and manage pollution.

68. START HARMONIZING YOUR ENVIRONMENT

The simplest method for reducing radiation is to remove all electric and electronic items out of your bedroom. Secondly, do some outdoor barefoot walking or sit outside on sand, grass or natural rock on a regular basis. You can also get EMF protection necklaces, bracelets, grounding footwear, and EMF protection stickers for your cell phone, TV, DVD player, pc, laptop, electronic reading devices, kitchen appliances, etc. There are pluggable EMF protection units, both for electric outlets and USB ports. If you want to research this further browse keywords like EMF pollution protection, ormus, orgone, electromagnetic field energy, scalar energy, electric body, crystal energy balancing, bioacoustics, and bio-geometry.

69. STOP DRINKING BEVERAGES OTHER THAN PURE WATER

Water is essential to life and is necessary for the body to rid itself of wastes and toxins. When you hear that one should drink a minimum of 8 glasses of pure water daily, it means exactly that: pure water. All other liquids don't count when calculating your daily intake of water. Liquid nutrient drinks like protein shakes, freshly pressed fruit or vegetable juices, fresh smoothies, fresh coconut water, and homemade soups are beneficial to your goal along with pure water and lemon water or water with lemon wedges. Some caffeine-free teas can be good for those who like tea. Any other beverages should be avoided. Industrially processed beverages should be excluded altogether.

70. DRINK FRESHLY PRESSED OR BLENDED FRUIT OR VEGETABLE JUICES

Try to drink a minimum of one glass of freshly pressed fruit of vegetables per day. You can combine any fruits or any vegetables, but don't mix fruits and vegetables. Some fruits cannot be juiced but can be blended. This includes bananas, avocados, and others. When juicing vegetables you will notice that very little juice comes out. Despite this it is best to juice vegetables because blending a bunch of vegetables might be a little too much indigestible fiber at once. You can also make vegetable soup and blend it before serving. That way, you will be able to digest tougher vegetables without a problem. Fresh juices help the body detoxify wastes and toxins and provide you with a massive amount of immediately usable nutrients.

71. TROPICAL FRUIT
Organic tropical and subtropical fruits like citrus fruits, pineapple, papaya, mango, kiwi, lychee, guava, persimmon, pomegranate, and others are beneficial for weight loss. Switching to real food will initially cause you to crave sweets and other sweetened junk foods. The process will be made easier with fresh fruits, freshly pressed fruit juices, fresh fruit smoothies, as well as lemon water or, simply, water with lemon, and fruity protein shakes. Fresh fruit is known to help cleanse the body, which, in turn, accelerates metabolism.

72. RAW ORGANIC UNFILTERED APPLE CIDER VINEGAR
Apple cider vinegar helps cleanse the body and use fat for energy. It stimulates digestion and improves pH balance. Consume a teaspoonful in a glass of water a couple of times per week after a meal.

CHAPTER FOUR: EXERCISE

73. STOP PROCRASTINATING WHEN IT COMES TO EXERCISE

Make exercise an essential part of your day, every day. Schedule time for exercise, be it a 4 minute stretching break, or a 4 hour sweat fest. The most important thing is that you develop the habit of exercising along with the habit of enjoying how good you feel afterwards.

74. UNDERSTAND THAT EXERCISE IS AN INSEPARABLE PART OF YOUR WEIGHT

Exercise is a phenomenal stress reliever and rejuvenator. Managing stress through exercise, among other methods, helps you get lean and stay that way because a less stressed state of mind equals less fat on your hips. Additionally, you burn more fat, digest your food better, eliminate wastes better, think better; and fit your clothes better.

75. STOP SPENDING ALL YOUR TIME SEATED OR STANDING

When we sit or stand for extended periods of time our circulation becomes stagnant, our metabolism slows, and we often suffer water retention. If you must sit or stand a lot do the following every hour or so for a minute or less:

get moving by walking around a little, bounce or jump, dance, shake, find an activity that requires whole body movement, go to the bathroom, step outside, stretch, march, do jumping jacks and squats, and whatever other movement comes to mind.

76. SPEND MORE TIME WALKING, DANCING, AND BOUNCING

Dedicate at least thirty minutes every other day to the above mentioned exercises. Also, spend at least fifteen minutes every other day doing focused stretching exercises or some basic yoga poses. Movement improves circulation and speeds up metabolism and fat burn. Stretching and yoga strengthen the body and the mind. Most types of exercise help you improve your ability to focus on your goals.

77. STOP SPENDING ALL YOUR TIME INDOORS

Indoor air leads to a lack of cellular oxygen, sluggish metabolism, low energy and motivation, and different health problems.

78. SPEND MORE TIME OUTSIDE

Oxygen and sunlight help oxygenate your cells, improve circulation, speed up metabolism, improve appetite and satiation, lift your mood, and help you stick with your goal. The body also obtains vitamin D from sunlight. Vitamin D supports overall health and hormonal balance. A stable weight and a healthy metabolism and muscle to fat ratio require your hormones to be in balance.

79. STOP WASTING TIME PRETENDING LIKE YOU ARE EXERCISING

Many people purchase a gym membership and do a bland version of exercise, spending half the time basically handing around in the gym. When exercising, you must have a plan and a strategy. You must want to learn something new on a regular basis and understand what exactly a specific type of exercise and a specific amount time or a specific tempo or the number of repetitions will do for you. Exercise is work and leisure at the same time. Study what you are doing by reading about it and talking to people about it. When you exercise, use your concentration and try your best to execute each exercise as well as you can. Observe how you feel during the exercise, immediately after the exercise, a couple of days after the exercise and after you have been doing the exercise for a couple of months, and so on. Keep an exercise diary and, again, write down how you feel, look and how your clothes fit you instead of the weight on the scale. The point is to do your best with the intention to feel your best.

CHAPTER FIVE: MINDSET

85. STOP TRYING TO LOOSE WEIGHT QUICKLY

Instead of focusing on losing weight, focus on getting lean. What this means is that you want muscle replacing fat. Fat is loose, muscle is dense. Fat is large and light, muscle is small and heavy. Forget the scale and focus on how you feel and how well your clothes fit and look on you. Focus on your energy and overall wellness. If you must lose weight, do so at a snail's pace, because if you do it fast you will lose muscle and you will not improve your muscle to fat ratio. If you want to be lean you must increase your muscle to fat ratio because it is muscle that burns fat and speeds up the metabolism. The body chemistry associated with a high muscle to fat ratio also helps prevent water retention. A high fat to muscle ratio does the opposite. It is a high muscle to fat ratio that keeps your hormones in balance (including your appetite and satiation hormones). A high fat to muscle to fat ratio does the opposite.

86. UNDERSTAND THAT YOUR WEIGHT IS AN INSEPARABLE PART OF YOUR LIFESTYLE

Your weight or more accurately your muscle to fat ratio is a direct reflection of your lifestyle.

80. LEARN TO VIEW YOUR EXERCISE SPACE AS YOUR PERSONAL BATTERY CHARGER

Most people today are stressed, overwhelmed and exhausted by everyday modern life. Time spent exercising can lift those feeling off your shoulders. Use it and be aware of its power, effectiveness and simplicity.

81. STOP BUYING THE BULL THAT A FEW MINUTES OF EXERCISE PER DAY WILL DO IT

If you exercise seven days a week you can have a few days a week on which you do mini exercise lasting less than 10 minutes each. That is, if you exercise for a minimum of 45 minutes the rest of the week. Ideally, exercise 45 minutes or more 3 days per week and up to 10 minutes 3-4 days per week. 175 minutes of total exercise time per week gives you an average of 25 minutes per day which is the ideal average and not something that requires taking away time from equally important things in your life. Combined with the consumption of exclusively real food (no industrially processed food) and some good, personalized supplements and effective time and stress management, you will have zero problems losing fat, strengthening your muscles and normalizing your weight. At a slow and steady pace, that is.

82. UNDERSTAND THAT LEAN MUSCLES COME FROM EXERTION

To have and maintain strong, lean muscles that will help you keep the fat off, you must practice resistance training. You must do exercises which force you to tighten your muscles to the maximum.

83. STOP THINKING THAT YOU CAN DO IT WITHOUT STRENUOUS EXERCISE

This can include lifting weights like free weights, weight lifting machines, certain ellipticals with arm presses, sprint running, lunge exercise with/without weights, various types of dance, winter sports, water sports, pilates, gymnastics, martial arts, etc. There are so many options that you will certainly find those which will appeal to you in the long run.

84. UNDERSTAND THAT RESISTANCE TRAINING WILL NOT TURN YOU INTO A GORILLA

Many women and some men fear that regular exercise and especially resistance training will make them look like brutes, men, monkeys, Rambo, etc. There may be one in a million individuals who possesses extraordinary tendencies to develop massive muscles, but most people must put in an enormous amount of work in order to achieve moderate results in terms of muscle mass. Most people who follow

the suggested program will simply look leaner with time until they have reached their genetic limit. Massive muscles or otherwise extremely defined musculature requires a special, personalized diet, lifestyle and exercise program. Most of all, it requires a high level of dedication and at least twice as much time invested per week in exercise alone.

80. LEARN TO VIEW YOUR EXERCISE SPACE AS YOUR PERSONAL BATTERY CHARGER

Most people today are stressed, overwhelmed and exhausted by everyday modern life. Time spent exercising can lift those feeling off your shoulders. Use it and be aware of its power, effectiveness and simplicity.

81. STOP BUYING THE BULL THAT A FEW MINUTES OF EXERCISE PER DAY WILL DO IT

If you exercise seven days a week you can have a few days a week on which you do mini exercise lasting less than 10 minutes each. That is, if you exercise for a minimum of 45 minutes the rest of the week. Ideally, exercise 45 minutes or more 3 days per week and up to 10 minutes 3-4 days per week. 175 minutes of total exercise time per week gives you an average of 25 minutes per day which is the ideal average and not something that requires taking away time from equally important things in your life. Combined with the consumption of exclusively real food (no industrially processed food) and some good, personalized supplements and effective time and stress management, you will have zero problems losing fat, strengthening your muscles and normalizing your weight. At a slow and steady pace, that is.

82. UNDERSTAND THAT LEAN MUSCLES COME FROM EXERTION

To have and maintain strong, lean muscles that will help you keep the fat off, you must practice resistance training. You must do exercises which force you to tighten your muscles to the maximum.

83. STOP THINKING THAT YOU CAN DO IT WITHOUT STRENUOUS EXERCISE

This can include lifting weights like free weights, weight lifting machines, certain ellipticals with arm presses, sprint running, lunge exercise with/without weights, various types of dance, winter sports, water sports, pilates, gymnastics, martial arts, etc. There are so many options that you will certainly find those which will appeal to you in the long run.

84. UNDERSTAND THAT RESISTANCE TRAINING WILL NOT TURN YOU INTO A GORILLA

Many women and some men fear that regular exercise and especially resistance training will make them look like brutes, men, monkeys, Rambo, etc. There may be one in a million individuals who possesses extraordinary tendencies to develop massive muscles, but most people must put in an enormous amount of work in order to achieve moderate results in terms of muscle mass. Most people who follow

64

the suggested program will simply look leaner
with time until they have reached their genetic
limit. Massive muscles or otherwise extremely
defined musculature requires a special,
personalized diet, lifestyle and exercise program.
Most of all, it requires a high level of dedication
and at least twice as much time invested per
week in exercise alone.

CHAPTER FIVE: MINDSET

85. STOP TRYING TO LOOSE WEIGHT QUICKLY

Instead of focusing on losing weight, focus on getting lean. What this means is that you want muscle replacing fat. Fat is loose, muscle is dense. Fat is large and light, muscle is small and heavy. Forget the scale and focus on how you feel and how well your clothes fit and look on you. Focus on your energy and overall wellness. If you must lose weight, do so at a snail's pace, because if you do it fast you will lose muscle and you will not improve your muscle to fat ratio. If you want to be lean you must increase your muscle to fat ratio because it is muscle that burns fat and speeds up the metabolism. The body chemistry associated with a high muscle to fat ratio also helps prevent water retention. A high fat to muscle ratio does the opposite. It is a high muscle to fat ratio that keeps your hormones in balance (including your appetite and satiation hormones). A high fat to muscle to fat ratio does the opposite.

86. UNDERSTAND THAT YOUR WEIGHT IS AN INSEPARABLE PART OF YOUR LIFESTYLE

Your weight or more accurately your muscle to fat ratio is a direct reflection of your lifestyle.

When you hear that you should eat healthy,
exercise and think positive, while it sounds
simplified, it is really true. Most importantly, it
is important that you understand and accept the
fact that in order to become and stay lean you
must optimize your lifestyle to an overall
satisfactory level. You cannot eat junk food, eat
irregularly, not pay attention to your digestive
regularity, not exercise, not pay attention to
your dietary needs, and not manage your stress,
and expect to look and feel your best.

87. STOP SPENDING TIME WITH PEOPLE WHO STRESS YOU OUT

Another source of stress is sometimes the
company we keep. If such company happens to
be the boss, review your reaction, perception
and interpretation of the negative impact. You
can either learn to diminish its importance or
find an acceptable approach for putting your
boss in his place or you can put your energy into
finding a more pleasant workplace. When it
comes to other types of relationships, take an
inventory and make a decision. The overall goal
here is to rethink your priorities and continue to
grow your stress management abilities.

88. START LIVING AND THINKING POSITIVELY

Enjoy the little things. Enjoy nature and
everything that it gives us. Expand your

consciousness and nurture your inner self.
Become positively aware of time and each
moment you can feel joy. It is your choice to feel
good and feel joy and bliss. This is your power.
Embrace it.

89. STOP BEING OVERWORKED

Start delegating, managing, organizing and
planning. Just like you must manage stress, you
must manage your time and your activities.
Again, rethink your priorities, make time for
yourself, take mini breaks, give others things to
do, and continue to improve your ability to focus
on the task at hand so as to save time without
hurry.

90. TAKE MINI BREAKS FROM LIFE: A MINUTE HERE, A MINUTE THERE

Make sure to take time out and not think of
anything you must do. Think of nothing or of
pleasant things. Anytime it is possible, spend
quiet time in nature and active time doing
outdoor exercises. Meditate, do slow, deep
breathing, do some bouncing, jumping or
dancing, or just have a laugh. Anything that is
not on your list of duties. Pretend that, for a
moment, you are on vacation.

91. STOP WORRYING AND STRESSING

Stress and worry cause the body to store more
fat and lead to cravings for fattening foods,

circulatory and digestive problems, and
metabolic and hormonal imbalances.

92. SPEND MORE TIME EXERCISING AND MEDITATING

Exercise can include any type of fun movement,
preferably outdoors or in a well aired space.
Discover a number of different types of
pleasurable physical activity and make it a habit
without overdoing it. You are looking to balance
your muscle to fat ratio and you will benefit from
extending that balance to all things. Meditation
can be traditional meditation or short naps,
daydreaming, visualization of your lean body
and related experiences, aerobic exercise,
stretching, yoga, dance, weight lifting, crossword
puzzles, and anything that is simultaneously
health supportive and relaxing.

93. STOP WASTING TIME ON UNPRODUCTIVE ACTIVITIES

Review your daily activities and discontinue
those which prevent you from being or staying
lean. This can include things that place
unnecessary stress on your mind/body/soul.
What you want is to get rid of the clutter, things
which waste your time and energy.

94. DEDICATE MORE TIME AND ENERGY TO FULFILLING ACTIVITIES

Inner fulfillment is important if you want a lean body. A lean body is a healthy body, a body in balance. In order for the body to be in balance, your mind and spirit must be in balance as well. Start viewing and treating your body, mind and soul as one. This will help you approach your goal from a holistic perspective.

95. WHAT IS BEHIND YOUR WEIGHT PROBLEM

Put time aside to take an inward look at your wellbeing and state of mind. Are there things and/or people that make your life more difficult than it should be? Do you hold on to negative feelings, neglect your needs and wants, and feel drawn to negative habits? If so, start working on changes that will lead you to a better management of how and with whom you spend your time. Learn to let go of the negative and embrace the positive. Try to resolve any issues and get into a better state of being.

96. SELF LOVE

Many people lack self love and as a result don't treat themselves optimally. People consume substandard and otherwise damaging foods and other substances (incl. cigarettes, alcohol, and legal and illegal drugs). People overeat, eat their meals irregularly, eat at night, skip breakfast,

70

eat too few healthy foods and too many
unhealthy foods, don't exercise or exercise
irregularly, don't spend time outdoors, don't get
enough sleep, etc. Any such habits must be
corrected if you want a lean body. Eat right,
exercise regularly, get your sleep, stick with a
healthy schedule, and create a better balance
between your obligations and your needs. Seek
healthful fulfillment. Most of all, love the food
that loves you back.

97. PRACTIVE LETTING GO
Some things we encounter on a regular basis
cannot be changed immediately and must
therefore be tolerated. In such instances we
must learn to not be negatively affected by them.
This is difficult but not impossible. Controlling
our thoughts or, more accurately, learning to
choose our thoughts and, thereby, control how
such annoyances make us feel, is key to this
process. With time, we realize that we no longer
feel as upset as we used to feel. Annoyances in
such instances represent a form of stress and,
as mentioned, we must actively learn to manage
stress.

98. LAUGHTER
It has been said that laughter is the best
medicine. Well, the next time you think of
industrially processed food, laugh at yourself.
You will notice that laughing feels better than

whatever industrially processed food you just felt you desperately needed. What you really needed was pleasure, something fun. And just like laughter makes you feel good, you will remember, over time, that there are many other pleasurable, fun things you enjoy immensely more than an edible factory product.

99. HOW BAD DO YOU WANT IT?
It is very important to raise this question because a decision must be made to change one's diet and lifestyle. Make the decision, use the tips, and make it happen.

100. MENTAL FOCUS
The final step on the list is about setting your mind for success. This means making the decision to get lean and stay lean indefinitely. It means changing your diet and lifestyle for good and giving your body as much time as it needs to reach that goal by forgetting that such a thing as a scale even exists. All you need to do is make the suggested changes and always keep your goal in your thoughts as if you are already there, because you have already placed yourself on that path by reading this book.

REFERENCES

OVERVIEW

Obesity Statistics
http://www.worldometers.info/obesity/
Study: World is getting fatter, needs to stop
http://thechart.blogs.cnn.com/2011/08/25/study-world-is-getting-fatter-needs-to-stop/
When Diet and Exercise are Not Enough: Roadblocks to Weight Loss
http://www.liveto110.com/when-diet-and-exercise-are-not-enough-roadblocks-to-weight-loss/
I Eat Real Food, Why Can't I Lose Weight?!
http://kellythekitchenkop.com/2011/07/i-eat-real-food-why-cant-i-lose-weight.html
Toxic Food Environment
http://www.hsph.harvard.edu/obesity-prevention-source/obesity-causes/food-environment-and-obesity/
The ability to eat cheaper home-cooked meals more often might explain why people appear to spend less money after retirement
http://blogs.lse.ac.uk/europpblog/2013/06/27/the-ability-to-eat-cheaper-home-cooked-meals-more-often-might-explain-why-people-appear-to-spend-less-money-after-retirement/
The Benefits of Growing Your Own Food
http://www.sparkpeople.com/resource/nutrition_articles.asp?id=1275

The Cooking Crisis: How to Get People Off the Couch and Into the Kitchen?
http://kathleenflinn.com/2011/09/26/how-do-you-get-people-off-the-couch-and-into-the-kitchen/

GRAINS & LEGUMES

Why Grains Are Unhealthy
http://www.marksdailyapple.com/why-grains-are-unhealthy/#axzz2cmznRg6H
The Real Truth About Those "Healthy Whole Grains"
http://www.realfooduniversity.com/real-truth-healthy-grains/
What's so bad about Grains?
http://www.cleanfoodcreativefitness.com/whats-so-bad-about-grains/
How Grains Are Killing You Slowly
http://wellnessmama.com/575/how-grains-are-killing-you-slowly/
Lectins and Fat Metabolism
http://weightgainblog.info/463/lectins-and-fat-metabolism/
Are You Eating These 3 Fat Gain Foods?
http://www.bradgouthrofitness.com/are-you-eating-these-3-fat-gain-foods/
Is Soy Making You Fat?
http://dustinmaherfitness.com/2009/07/is-soy-making-you-fat/
EMERGING DANGERS OF SOY PRODUCTS - by Sally Fallon and Mary Enig PhD
http://www.whale.to/a/fallon1.html

What is gluten? What is gliadin?
http://www.celiac.com/articles/8/1/What-is-gluten-What-is-gliadin/Page1.html

List Of Legumes
http://www.nourishinteractive.com/healthy-living/free-nutrition-articles/120-list-legumes

CANNED FOOD

Canned vs. Fresh Fruits and Vegetables
http://www.fitday.com/fitness-articles/nutrition/healthy-eating/canned-vs-fresh-fruits-and-vegetables.html#b

Avoiding Canned Foods and Drinks
http://www.shavernaturalmedicine.com/index.php/health-alerts/148-avoiding-canned-foods-and-drinks

Everyday metal toxicity in food
http://www.dnaindia.com/lifestyle/1822863/column-everyday-metal-toxicity-in-food

Canned Foods Health Risks - Chemicals Leach from Canned Foods
http://www.thedailygreen.com/healthy-eating/eat-safe/canned-foods-leach-chemicals-0330#slide-5

INFLAMMATION

Inflammation is a major reason why you can't lose weight
http://www.naturalnews.com/036701_inflammation_weight_loss_food.html

Inflammation: How to Cool the Fire Inside You That's Making You Fat and Diseased
http://drhyman.com/blog/2012/01/27/inflammation-how-to-cool-the-fire-inside-you-thats-making-you-fat-and-diseased/
Foods That Cause Inflammation and Promote Weight Gain
http://www.tracidmitchell.com/food/what-can-cause-weight-gain/

SWEETENERS

Artificial sweeteners: sugar-free, but at what cost?
http://www.health.harvard.edu/blog/artificial-sweeteners-sugar-free-but-at-what-cost-201207165030
Top 4 Most Dangerous Artificial Sweeteners
http://www.fitday.com/fitness-articles/nutrition/healthy-eating/top-number-most-dangerous-artificial-sweeteners.html#b
Diet Soda Health Risks: Study Says Artificial Sweeteners May Cause Weight Gain, Deadly Diseases
http://www.huffingtonpost.com/2013/07/11/diet-soda-health-risks_n_3581842.html
The Truth About Evaporated Cane Juice
http://www.processedfreeamerica.org/resources/health-news/405-the-truth-about-evaporated-cane-juice
"Sugar in the Raw" That's Not
http://www.thehealthyhomeeconomist.com/sugar-in-the-raw-thats-not/

76

Organic Sucanat
http://www.wholesomesweeteners.com/Products/pr
oductdetail/tabid/170/PId/8/Organic-Sucanat.aspx
8 Uses for Organic Beeswax
http://www.globalhealingcenter.com/natural-
health/beeswax/
Straight from the hive
http://www.reallyrawhoney.com/

BREAD STUFF ALTERNATIVES

Crackers and Breads
http://www.rawmazing.com/category/recipes/raw-
crackers-and-breads/
Home Made Raw Crackers!
http://theveganproject.ca/home-made-raw-
crackers/
Basic raw cracker recipe
http://www.therawtarian.com/basic-raw-cracker-
recipe
Crackers
http://nouveauraw.com/raw-recipies/crackers/
101 Dehydrator Recipes: Raw Flax Crackers
http://www.nourishingtreasures.com/index.php/20
12/10/11/101-dehydrator-recipes-raw-flax-
crackers/
Raw Flax Crackers Recipe
http://www.eatingvibrantly.com/raw-flax-crackers/
Breads, Crackers, and Wraps
http://www.choosingraw.com/recipes/breads-
crackers-and-wraps/

Flaxseed Crackers Recipe - Raw Vegan Hummus Recipe
http://www.thedailygreen.com/healthy-eating/recipes/flaxseed-crackers-hummus-recipe
Vegan Raw Crackers/Breads/Wraps
http://pinterest.com/Vegantempo/vegan-raw-crackers-breads-wraps/

PROTEIN

Undenatured Whey Protein vs Whey Protein Isolate
http://paleohacks.com/questions/31614/undenatured-whey-protein-vs-whey-protein-isolate#axzz2cneZG46w
High-protein diet reduces appetite
http://www.nature.com/news/2006/060904/full/news060904-3.html
Eat Wild
http://www.eatwild.com/

FAT

The Skinny on Fats
http://www.westonaprice.org/know-your-fats/skinny-on-fats
WE ARE HEALTHY BECAUSE WE EAT LARD!
http://willwinter.com/articles/health-and-nutrition/we-are-healthy-because-we-eat-lard/

OILS

Unfiltered olive oil
http://www.antoniocelentano.com/images/250%20
ml%20bright%20large.jpg
Coconut Oil: 10 Uses for this Miracle Elixir
http://www.myfitnesspal.com/blog/McKayMachina/
view/coconut-oil-10-uses-for-this-miracle-elixir-
88556
Coconut Research Center
http://www.coconutresearchcenter.org/
3 Ways to Make Virgin Coconut Oil
http://www.wikihow.com/Make-Virgin-Coconut-Oil
Process line for obtaining avocado oil
http://www.westfalia-
separator.com/applications/renewable-
resources/avocado-oil.html
Grapeseed Oil Goodness
http://mountainroseblog.com/grapeseed-goodness/

SPICES

Real Salt
http://realsalt.com/
**All natural spices, herbs, blends, soups and
extracts**
http://spicehunter.com/
Bulk organic herbs, spices & essential oils
http://www.mountainroseherbs.com/index2.php
13 Spices That Help You Lose Weight
http://www.fitbie.com/eat-right/13-spices-help-you-
lose-weight
List of Indian spices
http://en.wikipedia.org/wiki/List_of_Indian_spices

Spice
http://en.wikipedia.org/wiki/Spice

VEGETABLES

List of root vegetables
http://en.wikipedia.org/wiki/List_of_root_vegetables
Cruciferous vegetables
http://en.wikipedia.org/wiki/Cruciferous_vegetables
#List_of_cruciferous_vegetables
Cruciferous vegetables
http://en.wikipedia.org/wiki/Cruciferous_vegetables
#List_of_cruciferous_vegetables
Lettuce Varieties: A Guide To What's What
http://www.huffingtonpost.com/2012/06/25/lettuc
e-varieties_n_1626023.html
Lettuce
http://en.wikipedia.org/wiki/Lettuce
Tips to grow your own lettuce garden
http://www.sheknows.com/home-and-
gardening/articles/952893/tips-to-grow-your-own-
lettuce-garden
Complete List Of Vegetables By Season
http://www.nourishinteractive.com/healthy-
living/free-nutrition-articles/98-vegetables-by-
season
List of culinary vegetables
http://en.wikipedia.org/wiki/List_of_culinary_vegeta
bles#Fruits
Green Pasture Blog
http://www.greenpasture.org/public/Blog/index.cf
m

FRUITS

List of culinary fruits
http://en.wikipedia.org/wiki/List_of_culinary_fruits
Tropical fruits & subtropical fruits
http://www.faculty.ucr.edu/~legneref/botany/trofruit.htm
Citrus
http://en.wikipedia.org/wiki/Citrus
Benefits of Drinking Lemon Water & How To Make Lemon Water
http://www.bradgouthrofitness.com/take-the-28-day-lemon-water-challenge/
Apple Cider Vinegar Health Benefits – Clear Skin, Weight Loss, Detox
http://www.eatingbirdfood.com/2012/02/health-benefits-of-apple-cider-vinegar-acv/
8 Amazing Uses for Apple Cider Vinegar
http://gerson.org/gerpress/8-amazing-uses-for-apple-cider-vinegar/

NUTS

Raw cheesecake recipe
http://www.therawtarian.com/raw-cheesecake-recipe
The Benefits of Soaking Nuts and Seeds
http://foodmatters.tv/articles-1/the-benefits-of-soaking-nuts-and-seeds
Eat This: Chestnuts
http://paleodietlifestyle.com/eat-this-chestnuts/
Nut (fruit)
http://en.wikipedia.org/wiki/Nut_(fruit)

DAIRY ALTERNATIVES

Hemp milk
http://en.wikipedia.org/wiki/Hemp_milk
Swedes Consuming Low-Fat Dairy Products Gain More Weight!
http://www.dietdoctor.com/swedes-consuming-low-fat-dairy-products-gain-moreweight
Could A Dairy Allergy Be Your Weight Gain Culprit?
http://www.organicauthority.com/health/could-you-lose-weight-on-the-anti-allergy-diet.html
Can hidden food or dairy allergies cause weight gain?
http://www.troyrecord.com/articles/2013/04/15/news/doc516bf5a19ba49378019347.txt
Dr. Oz: Learn if dairy causes weight gain, IBS, fatigue with 28-day challenge
http://www.examiner.com/article/dr-oz-learn-if-dairy-causes-weight-gain-ibs-fatigue-with-28-day-challenge
No More Bloating or Water Retention
http://www.dietcoachjudy.com/articles.php?id=166
Government Under Fire as Radiation Is Found in Milk, Rain
https://www.baycitizen.org/news/environmental-health/government-under-fire-radiation-milk/
Canada's Land of Milk and Strontium 90
http://www.enviroreporter.com/2013/02/canadas-land-of-milk-and-strontium-90/all/1/
Shopping Guide to Avoiding Organic Foods with Carrageenan
http://www.cornucopia.org/shopping-guide-to-avoiding-organic-foods-with-carrageenan/

82

Does Your Coconut or Almond Milk Contain a Known Carcinogen? Mine Does.
http://www.happy-mothering.com/05/health-2/nutrition-health-2/carrageenen-carcinogen-coconut-almond-milk/

Buy Tempt Hempmilk, a powerhouse of hemp nutrition
http://www.livingharvest.com/products/milk

Organic Unshelled (Whole) Hemp Seeds
http://www.happilyraw.com/hemp-seeds-whole--unshelled---organic-979-p.asp

Coconut Butter: Here's everything you need to know!
http://chocolatecoveredkatie.com/2012/06/30/coconut-butter-and-coconut-oil/

How to Make Raw Coconut Yogurt
http://healthnutnation.com/2013/04/02/how-to-make-raw-coconut-yogurt/

Homemade Coconut Milk... The Easy Way
http://www.rubiesandradishes.com/2013/05/13/homemade-coconut-milk-the-easy-way/

Flaxseeds Health Benefits
http://www.whfoods.com/genpage.php?tname=foodspice&dbid=81

How to make your own Raw Coconut Milk & Coconut Powder
http://kitchen-apparel.com/2/post/2013/01/how-to-make-your-own-raw-coconut-milk-coconut-powder.html

Homemade Flax Milk
http://www.healthfulpursuit.com/2012/04/homemade-flax-milk/

The Health Benefits of Hemp Seeds
http://cleancuisineandmore.com/health-benefits-of-hemp-seeds/
Nutty about chestnut milk
http://www.vegsource.com/talk/recipes/messages/100051279.html
Sweet chestnut milk
http://www.rawfoodrecipes.co.uk/Recipes%202/Nut%20milk/Sweet%20Chestnut%20milk.htm

FERMENTED FOODS

List of Fermented Foods & Vegetables that Can Heal Your Gut
http://articles.mercola.com/sites/articles/archive/2012/03/18/mcbride-and-barringer-interview.aspx
Health Benefits of Raw & Fermented Foods
http://www.foodrenegade.com/health-benefits-of-raw-fermented-foods/
Fermented & Raw
http://www.foodrenegade.com/the-basics/fermented-raw/
Fermented Foods Can Heal Your Gut and Make Your Skin Glow
http://www.youngandraw.com/fermented-foods-can-heal-your-gut-and-make-your-skin-glow/
Raw Fermented Recipes
http://www.rawfoodrecipes.com/recipes/category/fermented.html
Raw Fermented Foods
http://pinterest.com/beccamia4/raw-fermented-foods/

84

How to Make Homemade Vegan Lacto Fermented Veggies
http://www.choosingraw.com/how-to-make-homemade-vegan-lacto-fermented-veggies/

What is lacto-fermentation?
http://www.pickl-it.com/faq/102/what-is-lacto-fermentation/

Fermentation in food processing
http://en.wikipedia.org/wiki/Fermentation_in_food_processing

Your Guide to Making Raw Young Coconut Kefir
http://rawglow.com/blog/2009/08/15/your-guide-to-making-raw-coconut-kefir/

Fermentation Blog
http://www.wildfermentation.com/fermentation-blog/

Fermentation of cacao beans
http://www.cacaoweb.net/cacao-beans.html

SUPERFOODS

Powder Pure
http://powderpure.com/science/

Superfood rich in chlorophyll
http://greensplus.com/index.php/cPath/94

ORAC Green SuperFood
http://amazinggrass.com/product_info/7286/ORAC-Green-SuperFood-.html

Live Juice Powders
http://www.livejuicepowders.com/faq.php

Garden of Life's Blog
http://www.gardenoflife.com/blog

85

The Top 10 Best Superfoods to Include in Your Diet
http://articles.mercola.com/sites/articles/archive/2011/09/10/top-ten-best-superfoods.aspx
Top 6 Super Foods!
http://www.thebestofrawfood.com/super-foods.html
Top 10 Super Foods for Raw Vegan Diet
http://www.peak-health-now.com/10_super_foods_raw_vegan.html
Does Maca make you lose weight
http://paleohacks.com/questions/56633/does-maca-make-you-lose-weight#axzz2d9YcDqgN
The Benefits Of Maca Root Supplementation for Athletes and Bodybuilders
http://www.muscle-health-fitness.com/benefits-of-maca-root.html/
Maca ~ Natural Viagra for Women ~ Hormonal Balance and Rejuvenation
http://youtu.be/zPnSXu0nPg0
Maca Powder
http://livesuperfoods.com/live-superfoods-maca-powder.html
Maca news, articles and information
http://www.naturalnews.com/maca.html
How to Use Maca Root
http://www.macarecipes.com/

SUPPLEMENTS

Phyllis A. Balch: Books, Biography, Blog, Audiobooks, Kindle
http://www.amazon.com/Phyllis-A.-Balch/e/B000APEVQO

Chromium
http://www.whfoods.com/genpage.php?tname=nutri
ent&dbid=51
Trace Minerals Research
http://www.traceminerals.com/research/misc-
articles
Eidon Ionic Minerals
http://eidon.com/health/category/health
Vitamin D
http://www.whfoods.com/genpage.php?tname=nutri
ent&dbid=110
**Lose Weight Naturally: How Vitamin D Impacts
Weight Loss**
http://comluv.com/lose-weight-naturally-vitamin-
impacts-weight-loss/
Arginine Helps Weight Loss & Cardio Health
http://www.wellnessresources.com/weight/articles/
arginine_helps_weight_loss_cardio_health/
7 Best Foods that Contain Arginine
http://www.3fatchicks.com/7-best-foods-that-
contain-arginine/
**Nutritional Comparison: Coriander (cilantro)
leaves, raw vs Parsley, raw**
http://skipthepie.org/vegetables-and-vegetable-
products/coriander-cilantro-leaves-raw/compared-
to/parsley-raw/
Arginine, Ornithine, Lysine & Weight Loss
http://www.livestrong.com/article/291471-arginine-
ornithine-lysine-weight-loss/
What Foods Help Your Body Produce L-Ornithine?
http://healthyeating.sfgate.com/foods-body-
produce-lornithine-1390.html
All About Carnitine
http://www.bodybuilding.com/fun/issa53.htm

87

Carnitine (L-carnitine)
http://umm.edu/health/medical/altmed/suppleme
nt/carnitine-lcarnitine
An In-Depth Analysis Of L-Tyrosine
http://www.bodybuilding.com/fun/md1.htm
**My Exhausting Search For More Energy and
Where I Finally Found It**
http://paleoonpaleo.com/paleo-thyroid-energy-
supplement/
L-glutamine And Weight Loss
http://www.livestrong.com/article/232707-l-
glutamine-and-weight-loss/
Glutamine
http://www.whfoods.com/genpage.php?tname=nutri
ent&dbid=122
Health Benefits of Conjugated Linoleic Acid
http://www.mercola.com/beef/cla.htm
**Scientific Proof That CLA Has Fat-Burning
Properties!**
http://www.bodybuilding.com/fun/david22.htm

CLEANSING

**Is your body being fooled into gaining weight by
xenoestrogens?**
http://www.naturesfare.com/blog/is-your-body-
being-fooled-into-gaining-weight-by-xenoestrogens-
by-brad-king/
The Benefits of Eating Seaweed
http://www.tidalgreens.com/benefit.html
SEAWEEDS USED AS HUMAN FOOD
http://www.fao.org/docrep/006/y4765e/y4765e0b.
htm

88

Edible seaweed
http://en.wikipedia.org/wiki/Edible_seaweed
Seaweed Health Benefits
http://www.thebestofrawfood.com/seaweed-health-benefits.html
Cyanobacteria
http://en.wikipedia.org/wiki/Cyanobacteria#Dietary_supplementation
Chlorella
http://en.wikipedia.org/wiki/Chlorella#Alternative_medicine
Edible Microalgae
http://www.ediblemicroalgae.com/intro/
Heavy Metal Detox Juice Recipe
http://www.mindbodygreen.com/0-9217/heavy-metal-detox-juice-recipe.html
How to Remove Heavy Metals from Your Body
http://life.gaiam.com/article/how-remove-heavy-metals-your-body
Detox Benefits (Heavy Metal Cleanse Benefits)
http://youtu.be/8-lFutB5QVo
Heavy Metal Toxicity and Detoxification Protocol
http://www.eidon.com/detox-protocol.html
Top foods that chelate the body of heavy metals
http://www.naturalnews.com/038670_heavy_metals_chelation_foods.html
Cilantro: Herb Assists in Heavy Metal Detoxification
http://www.naturalnews.com/027942_cilantro_heavy_metals.html
Spirulina and Chlorella Aid Heavy Metal Detox
http://www.naturalnews.com/027740_spirulina_chlorella.html

Chlorella: Detox Agent for Heavy Metals
http://articles.mercola.com/sites/articles/archive/2
013/01/28/chlorella-for-mercury-poisoning.aspx

Guide to Fresh Herbs: Recipes and Cooking
http://www.foodnetwork.com/recipes-and-
cooking/guide-to-fresh-herbs/index.html

Parsley
http://en.wikipedia.org/wiki/Parsley

Parsley
http://www.whfoods.com/genpage.php?tname=foods
pice&dbid=100

**Whole Body Detoxification (Part 3): Far-Infrared
Sauna Use**
http://www.naturalnews.com/022847_body_skin_de
toxification.html

**Dr. Brian Clement on Infrared Saunas and
Detoxification**
http://articles.mercola.com/sites/articles/archive/2
012/03/21/dr-clement-on-detoxification.aspx

9 Natural Remedies for Cellulite
http://wellnessmama.com/8608/9-natural-
remedies-for-cellulite/

How to Use a Wooden Massager on Cellulite
http://www.ehow.com/how_7414641_use-wooden-
massager-cellulite.html

Dry Brushing
http://drybrushing.net/

Dry Brushing: Benefits and Techniques
http://www.osmosis.com/post/1378407-dry-
brushing-benefits-and-techniques

**Lymphatic Drainage for the Legs - Self Massage
from MassageByHeather.com**
http://youtu.be/ZLyT_0Tr40M

Detox Your Liver with These Natural Herbs
http://www.naturalnews.com/027607_liver_detox_h
erbs.html

Kidney Cleanse – What You Need to Know
http://altmedicine.about.com/od/detoxcleansing/a/
kidney_cleanse.htm

How Probiotics Assist a Colon Cleansing Program
http://www.oxypowder.com/how-probiotics-assist-a-
colon-cleansing-program.html

Probiotics again linked to fat and weight loss: RCT data
http://www.nutraingredients-
usa.com/Research/Probiotics-again-linked-to-fat-
and-weight-loss-RCT-data

Take Probiotics To Lose The Belly Fat
http://www.charlespoliquin.com/ArticlesMultimedia
/Articles/Article/715/Take_Probiotics_To_Lose_The_
Belly_Fat.aspx

Consuming Probiotics Helps Overall Promote Healthy Digestive Function
http://www.brendawatson.com/Healthy-
Living/200811/Probiotics-and-Your-Health-Lifelong-
Partnership.htm

Busting the myths about probiotics and probiotic supplements
http://www.probiotic-myths.com/default.aspx

Digestive Enzymes Can Influence Weight Loss
http://voices.yahoo.com/digestive-enzymes-
influence-weight-loss-5633502.html?cat=68

Why You Should Take Systemic Enzymes - How to Build Muscle
http://jasonferruggia.com/why-you-should-take-
systemic-enzymes/

91

Everything You Learned about Enzymes was Wrong by Dr. William Wong
http://www.systemicenzymetherapy.com/TherapeuticApplications/Everything.htm
Enzyme FAQs
http://www.enzymedica.com/education/enzyme-faqs.html

EXERCISE

Physical exercise
http://en.wikipedia.org/wiki/Physical_exercise
Combat Conditioning: Five Months Without Weights!
http://www.bodybuilding.com/fun/mahler19.htm
What Muscles Do You Work On The Elliptical Machine?
http://www.livestrong.com/article/89981-muscles-work-elliptical-machine/
How To: Dumbbell Stepping Lunge
http://youtu.be/D7KaRcUTQeE
Basic Exercise Routine to Lose Weight
http://www.keepitmovingfitness.com/basic-exercise-routines/
11 Beginner's Yoga Poses To Help You Get Started
http://www.buzzfeed.com/mattortile/11-beginners-yoga-poses-to-help-you-get-started

SELF-FULFILLMENT

10 Keys to Inner Fulfillment
http://www.markbancroft.com/images/10_Keys_Inner_Fulfillment.pdf

Finding Inner Peace and Fulfillment
http://www.berzinarchives.com/web/en/archives/a
pproaching_buddhism/introduction/finding_inner_p
eace_fulfillment.html
How to Find Inner Fulfillment in Your Life
http://improve.mypkweb.com/how-to-find-inner-
fulfillment-in-your-life/
**Self-Love is Not a Crime: Learning to Love
Yourself**
http://psychcentral.com/blog/archives/2013/05/2
3/self-love-is-not-a-crime-learning-to-love-yourself/
**Learning Self-Love: 5 Tricks for Treating Yourself
More Kindly**
http://www.drchristinahibbert.com/5-tricks-for-
treating-yourself-more-kindly-increasing-self-love/
**21 Tips to Release Self-Neglect and Love Yourself
in Action**
http://tinybuddha.com/blog/21-tips-to-release-self-
neglect-and-love-yourself-in-action/
How to Love Your Authentic Self
http://tinybuddha.com/blog/how-to-love-your-
authentic-self/
**Laughter is the Best Medicine: The Health
Benefits of Humor**
http://www.helpguide.org/life/humor_laughter_heal
th.htm

AUTHOR

"100 Steps to a Lean Body" is my second book on the subject of wellness, after **"So Long Constipation, Part 1"**. Both books deal with seemingly minor wellness issues which affect most of us at some time or another. My third book on the subject of wellness will be a short one like **"100 Steps to a Lean Body"** and will be all about hormonal balance with an emphasis on testosterone. When I started writing **"100 Steps to a Lean Body"** I wasn't sure whether I would be able to squeeze in all the important info into a short book, considering that I managed to write over 500 pages on the subject of constipation in **"So Long Constipation, Part 1"**. Now I can see that I have achieved my goal and I am pretty happy with the resulting book. My hope is that as many people as possible feel inspired and motivated to achieve their wellness goals and continue to learn more on the subject. For questions or comments go to http://katarinanolte.com/.

Surprise bonus gift...

So Long

CONSTIPATION

PART 1

Katarina Nolte

Chapter One: Constipation

*Most people think that they are not constipated if they
are having one bowel movement a day. Yet, we eat
three meals a day. Where are the other two meals
going if they're not being eliminated through the colon?
The answer actually is somewhat frightening. The rest
of the food that is not absorbed by the body as
nutrients stays around the body in unlikely places --
against the colon walls, in tissues and organs, in
arteries -- any place at all in the body can serve as a
receptacle for uneliminated waste.*
Keeping your colon clean
http://www.naturalnews.com/033165_colon_cleansing_h
ealth.html

Cognizance

First, an estimated 90 percent of the population has a problem with candida overgrowth, although most don't know it.
Antibiotics Cause Cancer?
http://www.huffingtonpost.com/kim-evans/antibiotics-cause-cancer_b_186968.html

So Long Constipation, Part 1 is about much more than constipation. The reason is very simple: once you get rid of constipation you will not only want to remain constipation-free, but also continue to increase your newly regained wellbeing. This will take time and the willingness to learn more on the subject.

To be consistently successful on this road, it is best to try one thing at a time, and see how well it can be integrated into your lifestyle and schedule, as well as how it suits your individually unique mind-body chemistry. Regardless of the degree or frequency of the constipation and related ailments, it is important not to skip any parts of So Long Constipation, Part 1 that may not appear to apply and instead read this book in its entirety. Our bodies are not manmade engines which can be taken apart and repaired or replaced part by part. The human body, or the body of any mammal for that matter, is a complex system in which internal and external actions must work

97

in concert in order for us to function and feel our best, regardless of age and other factors. What we consume and how we consume it, along with our general awareness and attitude, are the most essential components of this process.

The more clearly we see the connection between consumption and function (or dysfunction), food and wellbeing, the more competent we become at replacing discomfort with wellness.

When it comes to constipation, one thing can lead to another, and before we know it, we realize that we are no longer enjoying optimal health. The constipation chain reaction can begin with the commonly known symptoms such as incomplete evacuation, straining, pain, discomfort, stools not passing easily, hard stools, dry stools, tiny stools, infrequent bowel movements, urge to go and then nothing, etc. This obvious failure to eliminate thoroughly can then lead to things like gas, cellulite, hernia, hemorrhoids, varicose veins, indigestion, weight gain, diverticulitis, insomnia, headaches, cancer, compacted fecal matter, bad breath, body odor, depression, fatigue, pain, abdominal cramps, bloating, weight gain, headaches, backaches, appendicitis, polyposis, neuropathy, megacolon, irritable bowel (IBS), inflammatory bowel disease (IBD), premenstrual syndrome (PMS), menstrual cramps, appendicitis, ulcers, chronic inflammation, internal bleeding, anal fissures,

98

etc. And it all begins due to the lack of knowledge, like what to eat and what to avoid, and that, ideally, one should have between one and five easy and smooth bowel movements every single day.

Did You Pop Today?
http://www.globalhealingcenter.com/constipation-and-colon-cleansing/poop
Constipation
http://en.wikipedia.org/wiki/Constipation
Constipation
http://digestive.niddk.nih.gov/ddiseases/pubs/constipation/
If you suffer from chronic or periodic constipation we have some pointers on how to have natural healthy regular bowel movements.
http://www.ageless.co.za/constipation.htm#Stress

Constipation rarely happens out of the blue in otherwise healthy adults. It is usually preceded by decades of semi-regular stools that are either too large, or too hard, or both. These abnormal stools cause gradual nerve damage and enlargement of the colon, rectum, and hemorrhoidal pads until one day the bowels refuse to move as was meant by nature — once or twice daily, usually after a meal, and with zero effort or notice.

Frequently Asked Questions: Constipation
http://www.gutsense.org/constipation/faq.html

Cradle to Grave

New research shows that soy oil makes for an amazing lubricant for skateboards or door hinges, while soybeans provide a fantastic insect repellent. Mosquitoes avoid it like the plague.
The selling of Frankensoy© What Doctors Don't Tell You
http://www.healthy.net/scr/article.aspx?Id=7746

Due to our typically unnatural diet and lifestyle, constipation is a slowly evolving dysfunction of the gastrointestinal system beginning in infancy and progressing as we age and is accompanied by other symptoms of digestive deterioration. The path from constipation to neurological degeneration includes malnutrition (nutrient-poor diet), malabsorption of nutrients, and toxin reabsorption (from stool). This is particularly devastating for infants and children whose growth and development depend on the amounts of nutrients they receive. Similarly, the aging population (40+) requires complete and proper digestion as their slowing systems struggle to maintain homeostasis.

One of the most important steps that must be taken in order to eliminate constipation for good is to revive our taste buds, which just like our olfactory (sense of smell) become desensitized when bombarded by artificial substances. While our sense of smell is weakened by industrial

100

perfumes, deodorants, deodorizers, etc., our
taste buds (and our olfactory system) suffer due
to exposure to pesticides, fungicides, herbicides,
additives (incl. flavors), colors and dyes, leading
to the inability to fully taste and enjoy natural
foods. The compromised taste and smell
functions distort our instinctive ability to crave
and choose foods our bodies need for optimal
function.

Further, our primal instincts are tricked by a
new, 5th 'taste' (fresh from the laboratory),
called 'umami' or 'savory'. It is the taste of none
other than monosodium glutamate (MSG),
commonly found in restaurant food, frozen
meals, dried meals, canned foods, and other
ready to eat preparations.

Aside from a truly natural diet, cleansing, once
again, is critical for the regeneration of the
senses as these require optimal function of our
various glands (along with the rest of the
internal system).

Digestive System
http://www.jonbarron.org/enzymes/digestive-health-acid-reflux-ulcers
Olfactory system
http://en.wikipedia.org/wiki/Olfactory_system
Umami
http://en.wikipedia.org/wiki/Umami
Frequently Asked Questions: Constipation
http://www.gutsense.org/constipation/faq.html
What Is The Connection Between Infant Constipation, Diarrhea, and Autism?
http://www.gutsense.org/constipation/autism.html

Do Artificial Flavors Spoil Us For the Taste of Real Food?
http://www.nytimes.com/1996/01/03/garden/do-artificial-flavors-spoil-us-for-the-taste-of-real-food.html
Flavor
https://en.wikipedia.org/wiki/Flavor

Up to 75% of what we perceive as taste is due to smell.
Digestive System
http://www.jonbarron.org/enzymes/digestive-health-acid-reflux-ulcers

Canal

It is really true that the mouth of a dog that drinks from the toilet is cleaner than yours. And if you must be bitten, better to be bitten by a dog than a person.
Digestive System
http://www.jonbarron.org/enzymes/digestive-health-acid-reflux-ulcers

Digestion begins in the nose, which alerts us to the presence of food and tells us what to eat. It continues in the mouth, where it is assisted by taste buds and enzyme-rich saliva. Expert opinion varies when it comes to the question of whether the human jaw is that of an omnivore (eats everything), a frugivore (mostly fruitarian), or a carnivore (mega meat lover).
From the mouth, food passes through the esophagus, and land in the stomach. Digestion

is assisted by the liver, kidneys, the gallbladder, the bile duct, and the pancreas.

Finally in the small intestine, nutrient absorption takes place with the help of beneficial gut bacteria and digestive enzymes. The rest of the content is indigestible stuff and includes metabolic waste, pharmaceuticals, heavy metals, and the various inedible factory food additives.

In addition, it is in the gut where stuff we absorb from water, air, and cosmetics, is processed and eliminated, which, in turn, makes digestive (gut cleansing) and extra-digestive (sweating, exercise, meditation) cleansing so crucial, along with a natural diet/lifestyle.

A healthy pancreas is crucial for optimal digestive functioning, because it is the pancreas that regulates blood sugar, and produces enzymes essential for proper digestion of food and the absorption of vital nutrients.

Industrially processed food overworks the pancreas, so that, over time, digestive and extradigestive health issues arise. These are: tummy ache, nausea, malabsorption, constipation, low energy, itchy skin, jaundice, cellular starvation, as well as diabetes and related cardiovascular and neurological problems.

Is It Your Stomach or Is It Your Pancreas That's Causing Pain?
http://www.NaturalNews.com/023161_pancreas_health_insulin.html

103

Digestive System
http://www.jonbarron.org/enzymes/digestive-health-acid-reflux-ulcers
Human as Frugivore
http://www.whale.to/a/frugivore_h.html
The Fruitarian Worldwide Network
http://www.fruitnet.org/

Sometimes after any type of abdominal surgery scar tissue will grow internally and pinch off or restrict a section of your bowel.
Did You Poop Today?
http://www.globalhealingcenter.com/constipation-and-colon-cleansing/poop

Missing

The Chinese did not eat unfermented soybean products.
THE PLOY OF SOY - Enzyme Inhibitors
http://www.consumerhealth.org/articles/display.cfm?ID=20000501001338

Chronic constipation often leads to high blood pressure and heart problems. Women are more likely to suffer from constipation and cardiovascular problems due to industrial toxins (air, water, food, and manmade products), anatomy (uterus), pregnancy, iatrogenic illness, chronic stress, lack of exercise, malabsorption, and nutritional deficiencies (enzymes, friendly gut bacteria, antioxidants, protein, magnesium, trace elements, and healthy oils).

Constipation can be caused by unforeseen events affecting the mind (unexpected event) or the entire mind-body system (travel, accident, etc.) in a stressful manner.

It can also be caused by industrially processed food, food allergies and intolerances, a sedentary lifestyle and consequential muscular weakness, pharmaceuticals, alcohol, anal sex, dry climate, and advanced age (70+).

Constipation can as well be a symptom of a given disease or a side effect of the treatment of a disease (surgery, anesthetics and other meds, colonoscopy, scar tissue, missing organs, radiation, etc.).

A less known type of constipation is caused by improper prioritization. Rather than going to the bathroom when we feel the urge, we postpone the deed, thereby training the body to discontinue bowel movement signaling. And then, when we finally go to the bathroom, nothing happens, causing the stool to linger and dry up, and making it difficult to expel the next time we do go to the bathroom when nature calls. Long term, this can cause chronic or even acute constipation.

People can also be constipated for no apparent reason. A general attitude that is on the restricted, restrained side due to unresolved

issues, can translate into repressed bodily
functioning.

Different Types of Constipation
http://www.articlesbase.com/alternative-medicine-
articles/different-types-of-constipation-588948.html

**Stress may take two paths in depression - endogenous
and reactive depression**
http://findarticles.com/p/articles/mi_m1200/is_n4_v146
/ai_15657596/

Is Constipation Stressing Your Heart Out?
http://recipetohealth.com/uncategorized/is-constipation-
stressing-your-heart-out-here%e2%80%99s-6-ways-to-
avoid-constipation/

Iatrogenic - Definition
http://www.thefreedictionary.com/iatrogenic

Death by Medicine–Iatrogenic illness
http://sustainablemedicine.org/2008/10/death-by-
medicine-iatrogenic-illness/

*Recognition of the psychosomatic factors that
influence the etiology of constipation. Finally,
psychology plays a huge role in constipation because
the very last act of moving the bowels — letting it go
— can be controlled and... suppressed at will. Sure,
the ability to withhold moving the bowels is an
absolutely essential trait for city dwellers, but,
unfortunately, taken too far, it is behind many cases
of chronic constipation.*

Frequently Asked Questions: Constipation
http://www.gutsense.org/constipation/faq.html

Spine

Constipation occurs when the waste material becomes blocked in the lower intestine. The blockage can cause pressure in the lower back. The pain will get worse if the impaction isn't eliminated. That's because your body continues to produce waste material even if it's not passing it. Conversely, back pain from lifting, a sudden jerk, or other straining activities can cause a bout of constipation. That's due to the fact that the muscles in the lower back in spasm can interfere with the autonomic nerves responsible for peristalsis of bowel movements.

Constipation and Back Pain
http://www.globalhealingcenter.com/back-pain-constipation.html

Constipation can cause back pain and vice versa. Both health issues are most common among women and people over the age of 30. Constipation is however not the sole culprit causing back pain, but rather the fact that constipated individuals' systems carry a backlog of metabolic wastes of all sorts. Most toxins have a neurotoxic effect raking havoc on the spinal part of the central nervous system, among other things. Additionally, a stuffed colon may be causing pressure, which results in back pain and discomfort. Excessive straining during difficult bowel movements can further exacerbate the situation, as can weak or

107

unbalanced muscles (back, buttocks, waist, hip, and abdominal muscles).

Back pain constipation is often related to mental-, spiritual-, or emotional stress which can be gradually alleviated with regular practice of relaxing activities like meditation, stretching, music therapy, dancing, aromatherapy, light therapy (preferably outdoors), walking and/or semi jogging (walk-jog-walk), and various types of nature therapy like gardening or hiking. Furthermore, slow tempo exercise leads to more intense deep tissue (muscle directly attached to bone) strengthening with less pressure on the joints/spine and an increased emphasis on posture and execution.

Back Pain Constipation
http://www.colon-cleanse-constipation.com/back-pain-constipation.html
Why Nature Is Therapeutic
http://www.wilderness-programs-info.com/nature-is-therapeutic.html
Fast vs Slow: Tempo demystified
http://theswole.com/general/fast-vs-slow/
Muscle weakness
http://en.wikipedia.org/wiki/Muscle_weakness
Spiritual Stress - Stress Management
http://www.netplaces.com/stress-management/what-is-stress-doing-to-me/stress-on-your-spirit.htm

Fiber is ok to digest as long as food does not contain too much of it. Unlike pigeons, we do not have a crop in which we can pre-digest cereals. And unlike cows, we do not have 4 stomachs to gradually ferment vegetables and grasses. Our bowels do not like

108

*excessive fiber. 'Foods' containing much fiber make
your bowels age much faster.*
Food Causing Constipation
http://www.13.waisays.com/constipation.htm

Roughage

*Environmental toxins modify our genes and affect our
children and grandchildren; enormous implications for
risk assessment of synthetic chemical and other
xenobiotics.*
Epigenetic Toxicology
http://www.i-sis.org.uk/epigeneticToxicology.php

The most important thing to know about fiber in
relation to constipation is that fiber is found in
plant foods, and that it is the plant foods that
are healthy for digestion, not the fiber per se.
This is because plant foods contain many other
health supporting nutrients, which together with
soluble (digestible) fiber stimulate proper
digestion. The popular idea of roughage solving
the problem of constipation is entirely incorrect,
as roughage tends to do the very opposite.
Many plant foods consist of both, soluble
(digestible) and insoluble (indigestible) fiber, and
should therefore be avoided until constipation
has been eliminated. Plants with indigestible
fiber are primarily those which require soaking
and/or cooking prior to consumption, like
grains, beans, corn, nuts, and seeds.

109

Indigestible parts of plant foods can damage the digestive function and microbial balance, leading to bloating, gas, indigestion, constipation, etc. Further, excessive consumption of starchy carbohydrates (grains, corn, beans, and rice) leads to excess fiber and blood sugar, which then lead to digestive-, weight-, and skin problems (as a starter).

And finally, one of the main reasons why roughage is a really bad idea when one is constipated is that it bulks up the stool which had a hard time passing to begin with. Cramps, discomfort, and exhaustion follow, due to the fact that fat absorption is compromised. Essential fat-soluble vitamins and minerals now cannot be utilized by the body. This malabsorption and malnutrition then lead to immunity-, endocrine-, cardiovascular-, connective tissue-, and weight problems.

People who suffer from constipation are often unable to digest many vegetables. In such cases, a balanced consumption of salad vegetables, cooked cruciferous veggies, and most of all freshly pressed fruit or vegetable juices, solves the problem.

Once again, the benefits of fiber are limited to soluble (digestible) fiber in combination with the countless nutrients found primarily in fresh, preferably organic, or at least local, fruits and vegetables.

110

Constipation is often either caused by, related to, or the cause of inflammation, which in turn aggravates some or all vital systems and functions. Fruits and vegetables, as well as freshly pressed juices thereof clear up the system, beat inflammation, and strengthen immunity, especially when consumed together with healthy fats (olive, coconut, fish, grape, and flax).

One of the consequences of eating inedible 'foods' like insoluble fiber, factory food (most of which is grain-, corn-, and/or soy-based), and laboratory spices (additives, preservatives, dyes, etc.), is the loss of healthy gut microbes, an overgrowth of unhealthy gut microbes, and an accumulation of metabolic wastes (undigested food, microbial waste products, etc.). Such a state, in turn, leads to an increase in inflammation and all types of ills and ails in the gut and beyond. The chaotically functioning gut will produce constipation, diarrhea, fungal infections, and autoimmune diseases.

An Apple a Day? Study Shows Soluble Fiber Boosts Immune System
http://www.sciencedaily.com/releases/2010/03/100302171531.htm

Dysbiosis
http://en.wikipedia.org/wiki/Dysbiosis

Dysbacteriosis-Symptoms and Treatment
http://intestinaldysbiosis.com/dysbiosis/dysbacteriosis-symptoms-and-treatment

Gut flora
http://en.wikipedia.org/wiki/Gut_flora

WHFoods: vitamin K
http://www.whfoods.com/genpage.php?tname=nutrient&
dbid=112
Coagulation
http://en.wikipedia.org/wiki/Coagulation
**Cut Down on Sugar and Carbohydrates to Improve
Health**
http://www.naturalnews.com/023343_sugar_food_carboh
ydrates.html
Do Carbohydrates Turn To Sugar In Your Body?
http://www.livestrong.com/article/505191-do-
carbohydrates-turn-to-sugar-in-your-body/
Dietary Fiber
http://en.wikipedia.org/wiki/Dietary_fiber
Cruciferous vegetables
http://en.wikipedia.org/wiki/Cruciferous_vegetables
**What are nightshades and in which foods are they
found?**
http://www.whfoods.com/genpage.php?tname=george&db
id=62

*Insoluble fiber produces hard-to-pass stools that can
distend and damage the intestinal lining, form
blockages of compacted food, and create anal
fissures. Excess soluble fiber creates massive
fermentation and prodigious amounts of gases, acids,
and alcohol, killing off the flora that normally hydrate
stools and prevent constipation.*

**Negative Implications: Rethink the Role of Dietary
Fiber**
http://www.naturalnews.com/029927_dietary_fiber_healt
h.html

Flames

Fiber doesn't keep [the] "colon clean" by speeding elimination, according to the highly respected and authoritative Rome II: The Functional Gastrointestinal Disorders textbook: "There is little or no relationship between dietary fiber and whole gut transit time." In fact, fiber delays transit time more than does any other food ingredient, and is the primary cause of chronic constipation, hemorrhoids, diverticulosis, ulcerative colitis, and Crohn's disease.

Fiber Menace: The Truth About the Leading Role of Fiber in Diet Failure, Constipation, Hemorrhoids, Irritable Bowel Syndrome, Ulcerative Colitis, Crohn's Disease, and Colon Cancer

http://www.amazon.com/Fiber-Menace-Constipation-Hemorrhoids-Ulcerative/dp/0970679645/

When gastrointestinal health is compromised, the rest of the body doesn't work as it should. Insoluble (indigestible) fiber ferments, forming gases, bloating, acidic wastes and intestinal inflammation, all of which disturb normal healing and regenerative processes.

If inflammation persists, becoming chronic, other imbalances occur, most frequently relating to blood sugar and insulin. Chronic inflammation leads to insulin resistance, which in turn causes diabetes, an exploding problem worldwide.

Chronic intestinal inflammation can cause belly fat accumulation (also related to blood sugar,

113

insulin, diabetes, and cardiovascular problems)
and depression, with researchers being unsure
which one comes first. What seems to be clear is
that it all begins with chronic inflammation,
which nowadays most commonly develops in the
digestive tract. Further, excess weight
compromises immunity, thereby prolonging
inflammation.

The primary cause of a chronically inflamed
digestive system is stress in the form of mental
and emotional stresses, and food, water, and air
compromised by industry.

**Type 2 Diabetes: Inflammation, Not Obesity, Cause of
Insulin Resistance**
http://www.sciencedaily.com/releases/2007/11/071106
133106.htm

Human gastrointestinal tract
http://en.wikipedia.org/wiki/Human_gastrointestinal_tra
ct#Immune_function

Diabetes becoming alarmingly common worldwide
http://www.washingtonpost.com/national/health-
science/diabetes-becoming-alarmingly-common-
worldwide-new-study-
finds/2011/06/24/AGMkaFlH_story.html

**Is Chronic Inflammation a Possible Cause of Obesity-
Related Depression?**
http://www.hindawi.com/journals/mi/2009/439107/

Inflammation
http://en.wikipedia.org/wiki/Inflammation#Systemic_infl
ammation_and_obesity

Gastrointestinal Diseases - Digestive System
http://www.diet-and-
health.net/Diseases/gastrointestinal.html

Uncomfortable digestive symptoms like bloating, gas, and bubbling in the gut arise because an overgrowth of yeast leads to the fermentation of foods instead of the digestion of foods. Along with these unpleasant symptoms, yeasts ferment sugars into alcohol, which destabilizes blood sugar and leads to intense cravings for more sugar. I find it fascinating that these tiny organisms can get us to do exactly what they want us to do — eat more carbs and sugar!

Yeast sensitivity, sugar cravings, and your digestion

http://www.womentowomen.com/digestionandgihealth/candida.aspx

Twist

Any health problems that compromise digestion and/or absorption of nutrients can contribute to deficiency of vitamin K. These problems include health conditions like inflammatory bowel disease, ulcerative colitis, celiac disease, short bowel syndrome, and digestive tract surgeries (like intestinal resection). Problems with pancreatic function, liver function, or gallbladder function can also increase our risk of vitamin K deficiency.

Because our intestinal bacteria help supply us with vitamin K, any drugs that alter our normal intestinal bacteria can compromise our vitamin K status. At the top of this drug list would be antibiotics.

What factors might contribute to a deficiency of vitamin K?

http://www.whfoods.com/genpage.php?tname=nutrient&dbid=112

115

Disproportionate amounts of fiber jeopardize the digestion of vital proteins, fats, vitamins, minerals, and trace elements, with the effect being connective tissue weakness, musculoskeletal problems, neurological damage, etc.

Grains, high in fiber, gluten, lectins, and phytates, disturb the balance of both, the digestive and the hormonal system, resulting in food cravings, overeating, cellular damage, stomach lining damage, and the appearance of the by now well known digestive conditions like irritable bowel (IBS), inflammatory bowel (IBD), Celiac, Crohn's, Candidiasis, leaky gut (LGS), etc.

The main problem with high fiber foods is that they are not meant for human consumption because they are too difficult to impossible to digest and were therefore originally soaked, sprouted, fermented, and/or marinated, so as to be made somewhat edible in moderate amounts. Unfortunately today, most people, regardless of where they live, use grains, corn, rice, and/or soy, as staple foods, thereby literally destroying their health and quality of life. To make matters worse, these and other foods are being increasingly genetically altered (GMOs) and exposed to poisonous substances originally invented to serve as weapons of war (pesticides, fungicides, herbicides, radiation, etc.).

As a result, children and adults suffer from the before mentioned digestive conditions along with, and related to malabsorption, malnutrition, autoimmune disease, and excess fat accumulations on and/or in the body (organ fat), with rotting, undigested food roaming freely and destroying vital organs and tissues.

The Lowdown On Lectins
http://www.marksdailyapple.com/lectins/
Lectins
http://en.wikipedia.org/wiki/Lectin
Essential Sugars and Plant Lectins
http://failsafediet.wordpress.com/about-food-chemical-intolerance/the-natural-toxins-in-food/essential-sugars-and-plant-lectins/
Why No Grains and Legumes? Part 1: Lectins
http://www.paleoplan.com/2011/03-30/why-no-grains-and-legumes/
What are nightshades and in which foods are they found?
http://www.whfoods.com/genpage.php?tname=george&dbid=62
FiberMenace: About the book
http://www.gutsense.org/fibermenace/about_fm.html
Cadaverine
http://en.wikipedia.org/wiki/Cadaverine
Diverticulosis and diverticulitis
http://www.gutsense.org/gutsense/diverticular.html
Why Grains Are Unhealthy
http://www.marksdailyapple.com/why-grains-are-unhealthy/#axzz1qa16Yvcq
Definitive Guide: The Primal Blueprint
http://www.marksdailyapple.com/definitive-guide-primal-blueprint/#axzz1qa16Yvcq

MAY I offer you some warm, bacteria-ridden dough topped with rotten milk and discs of rotten meat? No? That is a pepperoni pizza. If that sounds too unappetizing, substitute "bacteria-ridden" with "risen" (pizza crust, like bread, relies on the work of a unicellular fungus known as Saccharomyces cerevisiae—or, more commonly, yeast), and "rotten" with "fermented". The cheese and meat are both the delicious product of bacteria.

Fish sauce: The thin line between fermentation and rot
http://www.economist.com/blogs/prospero/2011/05/fish_sauce

Flurry

Prior to fermented products such as soy sauce, tempeh, natto, and miso, soy was considered sacred for its use in crop rotation as a method of fixing nitrogen. The plants would be plowed under to clear the field for food crops.

Soybean History
http://en.wikipedia.org/wiki/Soybean#History

Putrefaction (rotting) is done by microorganisms which impede digestion, nutrient absorption, and the elimination of wastes. Fermentation is done by microorganisms which support digestion, nutrient absorption, and the elimination of wastes.

Intentional fermentation has been practiced at least since the introduction of plant and animal

118

domestication, and in particular since humans begun consuming grains, corn, rice, beans, soybean, lentils, and peas.

Fermentation extends the shelf life of food, intensifies the taste and aroma of food, and makes food easier to digest by increasing the amount of healthy gut bacteria (in the food itself and in the gut post consumption).

Examples of fermented foods are: raw fermented dairy products (yogurt, kefir, sour cream; fresh and aged cheeses), raw fermented vegetables (sauerkraut, pickles); raw fermented eggs, meat, fish or seafood (liver-, fish-, or shrimp pâté; fish-, or oyster sauce; mayonnaise); raw fermented nuts and seeds (raw vegan "cheeses", pâtés, and sauces), fermented grains (soured porridge, kashk, trahanas, dhokla, naturally fermented breads and pastas), and fermented legumes (soy sauce, bean pâté, lactose-fermented lentils).

Constipation, as well as irritable bowel (IBS), inflammatory bowel disease (IBD), Crohn's, Candida, Celiac, leaky gut, etc., are all associated with insufficient amounts of friendly gut bacteria necessary for proper digestion. Therefore, naturally fermented foods may help some individuals replenish their flora.

Ideally, fermentation should be done at home, and one should stick with raw fermented foods, while avoiding grain-, soy-, and rice-based fermented foods and beverages.

119

Raw fermented foods offer a variety of flavors, are rich in enzymes, beneficial microorganisms, and vitamins, while cooking/pasteurization destroys them. Destruction of these vital substances, in turn, incapacitates the gut, exhausts the system, and leads to overall degeneration, including premature aging (example: adult diseases in children). Fermented fruit is a high fiber, high sugar alcoholic product, be it edible or drinkable. It should not be consumed by people who are constipated, or those who suffer from digestive conditions like irritable bowel (IBS), inflammatory bowel disease (IBD), Crohn's, Candida, Celiac, leaky gut, etc.

Probiotics are helpful digestive probiotic bacteria for Crohns
http://www.crohns.net/Miva/education/whatprobiotics.shtml

More Evidence Links Gut Bacteria to Celiac Disease
http://www.celiac.com/articles/21685/1/More-Evidence-Links-Gut-Bacteria-to-Celiac-Disease/Page1.html

Drunk Animals
http://www.metacafe.com/watch/90957/drunk_animals/

Poaceae
http://en.wikipedia.org/wiki/Poaceae#Taxonomy

Cereal
http://en.wikipedia.org/wiki/Cereal

Legume
http://en.wikipedia.org/wiki/Legume

Difference Between Fermenting and Rotting
http://www.superfoods-for-superhealth.com/Superfood_Evolution-fermented-food.html

120

Reflections on Rotten Food
http://chowhound.chow.com/topics/286173
8 Reasons to Eat Fermented Foods
http://www.cheeseslave.com/got-bacteria-10-reasons-to-eat-fermented-foods/
Raw Ferments - The Missing Link - The Forgotten Superfood
http://hiddenpondllc.com/content/4886
Injera
http://en.wikibooks.org/wiki/Cookbook:Injera
Kashk
http://en.wikipedia.org/wiki/Kashk
Tarhana
http://en.wikipedia.org/wiki/Tarhana
Why We Love Lactofermentation
http://cedarcirclefarm.org/tips/view/why-we-love-lactofermentation/
Would you eat fermented meat?
http://paleohacks.com/questions/11937/would-you-eat-fermented-meat#axzz1sAVhZjOg
High vs. Fermented Meat
http://www.rawpaleodietforum.com/general-discussion/high-vs-fermented-meat/
Fermented Foods
http://www.akealife.com/blueprint-for-life/nutrition/fermented-foods/
Fermented Eggplant Recipe
https://www.wholetraditions.com/recipes/124-fermented-eggplant
Carciofi Sott'Olio: Marinated Artichokes Recipe
http://www.foodnetwork.com/recipes/mario-batali/carciofi-sottolio-marinated-artichokes-recipe/index.html

Evidence has suggested that Dysbiosis plays a part in many conditions such as: Irritable Bowel Syndrome, Anklyosing Spondylitus, Rheumatoid Arthritis,

121

Inflammatory Bowel Disease, Multiple Sclerosis, Chronic Fatigue, Eczema, food allergies. Many people are unaware that they are even suffering from Dysbiosis.
Dysbiosis and Leaky Gut Syndrome
http://www.leakygut.co.uk/Dysbiosis.htm

Fire

It is erroneous to assume that any evidence of fire from millennia ago, must be of human origin, and then further jump to conclude that humans have been cooking for millions of years.
Advent of Cooking
http://www.rawpaleodiet.com/articles/dangers-of-cooked-foods-an-extensive-collection-of-on-and-offsite-articles/advent-of-cooking-article/

While natural fires in the form of volcanoes, lightning, and wildfires have been occurring over the past several hundred million years, research findings vary on the subject of when fire was first used by humans, and whether and when it has been used for the specific purpose of heating food. A similar disagreement exists on the question of when and how often humans created intentional fires, rather than taking advantage of accidental or natural fires on rare occasions. It is, of course, also not known to what extent foods were cooked, whether they were lightly steamed, smoked, or seared, etc., or whether the food was boiled or roasted for extended periods of time. The importance of these details lies in the fact that most people today experience digestive problems with regular consumption of overcooked and/or over processed foods. If our ancestors would have been consuming overwhelmingly cooked foods, our digestive systems would have an easy time processing such foods.

On the other hand, humans are the only animals who heat their food, so perhaps an adaptation is impossible. Pets which are fed mostly or exclusively processed foods (including foods cooked at home), tend to suffer from the same diseases as humans, when compared to pets whose diets consist of raw whole food (incl. bone, cartridge, internals, and outdoor plants, insects, etc.). The modern pet also tends to live half as long, on average.

Advent of Cooking
http://www.rawpaleodiet.com/articles/dangers-of-cooked-foods-an-extensive-collection-of-on-and-offsite-articles/advent-of-cooking-article/

Socializing around a campfire might actually be an essential aspect of what makes us human.
Humans Used Fire 1 Million Years Ago
http://news.discovery.com/human/human-ancestor-fire-120402.html

123

Jaws

Our teeth are brachydont, and aren't intended for chewing fiber, otherwise, after a decade or so, you simply wouldn't have any teeth left to argue this point with clarity. That's why the fiber for human consumption is crushed, milled, or ground first, and requires little or no chewing. But even after processing, it affects the oral cavity with a menacing vengeance.

Fiber Menace: Excerpts from the book

http://fibermenace.com/fibermenace/fm_chapter1.html

Parallel to the digestive tract being unable to handle processed foods, human jaws and teeth demonstrate the negative consequences of processed food consumption. The human jaw first shrunk when our archaic ancestors begun processing food by hand, and then once again since cooking was introduced, and again since the introduction of grains into the diet. Some believe that the shrinking of the human jaw, as well as the teeth, is ongoing because of the industrial revolution, the related spread of factory food products, and the ever increasing availability of portable, bite size food stuffs. This means that over the past couple of million years, humans reduced the frequency of biting into food (fruit, bugs, meat, roots, whole animals), followed by less chewing of raw foods (enzymes, friendly bacteria, and other

124

undenatured nutrients), and a gradual increase in the amount of grinding crunchy, chewy, sticky grain-based products and processed grain-fed animal products.

As a result and unlike (other) animals, humans have jaws that often cannot accommodate all 32 teeth, which then are misaligned, maloccluded, and rotting away (caries), while the jaw degenerates (gingivitis, periodontitis). Studies show that tribal children outside of civilization tend to develop perfectly matching sets of teeth as long as they don't consume factory foods. If they do, a mismatched development of jaw size and shape relative to teeth size and shape occurs and is followed by decay, gum disease and tooth loss later in life.

Human 'dental chaos' linked to evolution of cooking
http://www.newscientist.com/article/dn7035
Dangers of Cooked Foods
http://www.rawpaleodiet.com/articles/dangers-of-cooked-foods-an-extensive-collection-of-on-and-offsite-articles/
Toxins created by cooking
http://www.rawfoodlife.com/Articles__Research/Toxins_Created_by_Cooking/toxins_created_by_cooking.html
Epigenetics, DNA: How You Can Change Your Genes, Destiny
http://www.time.com/time/magazine/article/0,9171,1952313,00.html

The only body parts requiring regular surgery are the teeth.
Human 'dental chaos' linked to evolution of cooking
http://www.newscientist.com/article/dn7035

Brainy

*Dietary fat is the only substance that initiates the
action that precedes bowel movements.*
Frequently Asked Questions: Constipation
http://www.gutsense.org/constipation/faq.html

Between 3 million years ago and up until about
10,000-20,000 years ago, the average human
brain increased in size in proportion to the
increase in animal protein consumption (eggs,
meat, seafood, fish, sea animals, and poultry).
Among countless nutrients, the named animal
products provided humans with high levels of
healthy fats essential for thriving brains.
Presently it is known that inadequate amounts
of healthy fats in the diet lead to an array of
degenerative diseases, including serious
digestive-, neurological- cardiovascular-, and
musculoskeletal issues.
Toward the end of the last ice age, hunters ran
out of game and began eating what basically
amounts to indigestible grass seeds (grains).
Mass hunting involved enclosure, also known as
corralling, during which hunters would
surround large numbers of animals, and
slaughter them as they moved inward into the
center of the herd until all animals were dead.
Eventually, instead of killing all animals,
humans begun collecting the young, taming

126

them by providing nutrition and safety, and animal domestication was born.

What followed was the consumption of domesticated plants and animals, which are of inferior nutritional quality when compared to wild plants and animals. The agricultural lifestyle required a previously unheard of workforce, which in turn lead to more offspring being produced. The combination of chronic malnutrition, excessive reproduction, resource based war, and socioeconomic stratification over the past 10,000 years caused the human brain (skull) and body to weaken and shrink.

The more recent industrial revolution changed this somewhat for the better, but overall, our ancestors like the archaic Homo Sapiens and Homo Sapiens Neanderthalensis continue to represent the most robust humans with the largest skulls to date.

Quaternary extinction event
http://en.wikipedia.org/wiki/Quaternary_extinction_event

Civilization
http://en.wikipedia.org/wiki/Civilization

If Modern Humans Are So Smart, Why Are Our Brains Shrinking?
http://discovermagazine.com/2010/sep/25-modern-humans-smart-why-brain-shrinking

Big Brain: The Origins and Future of Human Intelligence
http://www.amazon.com/Big-Brain-Origins-Future-Intelligence/dp/1403979782

Neanderthals More Intelligent Than Thought
http://news.discovery.com/history/neanderthals-more-intelligent-than-thought.html
All Non-Africans Part Neanderthal, Genetics Confirm
http://news.discovery.com/human/genetics-neanderthal-110718.html
Asian Neanderthals, Humans Mated
http://news.discovery.com/history/neanderthal-human-mating.html
Sex with Neanderthals Made Us Stronger
http://news.discovery.com/human/neanderthals-interbreeding-humans-110825.html
Neanderthal Children Were Large, Sturdy
http://news.discovery.com/history/neanderthal-baby-teeth-family.html
Neanderthal Males Had Popeye-Like Arms
http://news.discovery.com/history/neanderthal-hormones-strong-arms.html
Advent of Cooking
http://www.rawpaleodiet.com/articles/dangers-of-cooked-foods-an-extensive-collection-of-on-and-offsite-articles/advent-of-cooking-article/

Brain-size has decreased by 8% since the advent of the Agricultural Revolution, which coincided with a massive increase in the consumption of cooked starchy foods... An increase in cooked starches, grains and the introduction of dairy to the human diet, coupled with a decrease in meat has caused great detriment to our species.
Advent of Cooking
http://www.rawpaleodiet.com/articles/dangers-of-cooked-foods-an-extensive-collection-of-on-and-offsite-articles/advent-of-cooking-article/

Captivity

Over the past 20,000 years, the average volume of the human male brain has decreased from 1,500 cubic centimeters to 1,350 cc, losing a chunk the size of a tennis ball. The female brain has shrunk by about the same proportion. If our brain keeps dwindling at that rate over the next 20,000 years, it will start to approach the size of that found in Homo erectus, a relative that lived half a million years ago and had a brain volume of only 1,100 cc.

If Modern Humans Are So Smart, Why Are Our Brains Shrinking?

http://discovermagazine.com/2010/sep/25-modern-humans-smart-why-brain-shrinking

The domestication of farm animals has lead to the domestication of humans themselves. Just like cattle and sheep, humans adapted by passing on decision making to whoever had power over food and food choices, the plain order of civilization.

Instead of living in tiny close knit groups with no manmade territorial limits, humans now inhabited limited spaces with comparatively extremely large numbers of strangers. As a result, the autonomous independence of individuals living in the wild was replaced by duteous dependence of individuals living in a controlled environment. The artsy-craftsy skillfulness of the hunter-gatherer, or more accurately scavenger-gatherer-hunter, was

129

fading and so was the human intellect. Normally, brain and body develop and grow in proportion, but at the onset of agriculture, the skull no longer grew to full completion, something that has been observed in domesticated animals as well. These new juvenile-brained humans favored reproduction with less aggressive (physically and otherwise), more compliant mates. As a result, the average lifespan dropped from 35 (pre-agricultural Paleolithic Era) to 25 (agricultural Greco-Roman Era), conservatively.

Neurodegenerative disease related to our grain-based diet and unnatural lifestyle affects the digestive tract as much as it affects the function and longevity of our brains. The consequence of agricultural civilization was not only the shrinking of the brain over generations, but also the shrinking and overall deterioration of the brain over the course of a lifetime.

Age related brain shrinkage begins around age 25 and is unique to the human species. Other animals (inc. primates) do not show such a decline, and it can therefore be concluded that the difference between us and other animals is the fact that we consume a diet to which we thus far have been unable to adapt to, and that as a consequence, we evolve, develop, and age in an inferior mode.

The Incredible Shrinking Human Brain
http://news.sciencemag.org/sciencenow/2011/07/the-incredible-shrinking-human-b.html

Our Brains Are Shrinking. Are We Getting Dumber?
http://www.npr.org/2011/01/02/132591244/our-brains-are-shrinking-are-we-getting-dumber
Nutrition for intellect
http://www.dailymotion.com/video/xfqq52_nutrition-for-intellect_lifestyle
If Modern Humans Are So Smart, Why Are Our Brains Shrinking?
http://discovermagazine.com/2010/sep/25-modern-humans-smart-why-brain-shrinking
Rapid Uplift: Ancient People Were Smarter Than Us
http://suvratk.blogspot.com/2008/04/ancient-people-were-smarter-than-us.html
Big Brain: The Origins and Future of Human Intelligence
http://www.amazon.com/Big-Brain-Origins-Future-Intelligence/dp/1403979782

In class today we examined the development of agriculture and compared hunter-gatherers to early Neolithic farmers. As humans domesticated plants and animals, the plants and animals themselves change over time. Wild sheep and mountain goats get fatter, slower, dumber, and lose their balance.
Learning to Farm
http://mrguerriero.blogspot.com/2011/11/learning-to-farm.html

Denatured

I adhere to the philosophy that both the living organism and its enzymes are inhabited by a vital principle or life energy which is separate and distinct

131

*from caloric energy. The enzyme complex harbors a
protein carrier inhabited by a vital energy factor.*
Enzyme Nutrition by Dr. Edward Howell
http://www.amazon.com/Enzyme-Nutrition-Dr-Edward-
Howell/dp/0895292211/

When it comes to the gut, the brain, and other
vitals, ORAC (Oxygen Radical Absorbance
Capacity) levels in foods play a notable role.
Some of the highest ORAC foods are berries,
cacao, cloves, cinnamon, curry/turmeric, cumin,
mustard, flax, chia, ginger, and culinary herbs.
Industrially processed, cooked foods lack vital
nutrients, and are more or less packed with
artificial substances which the body has no use
for, and which it is often unable to eliminate.
Heating food over the maximum heating capacity
of topsoil (115 °F/46°C) by the sun destroys
enzymes, friendly bacteria (which causes mold to
flourish), many vitamins, minerals, and trace
elements. For this reason, industrially processed
and/or overheated food has been given the term
'denatured' by people who consume foods with a
focus on nutritional value, and enzyme activity
in particular (raw-, paleo-, instinctive-, and local
foodists, vegans, and vegetarians).
Denatured or 'dead' food tends to do the
opposite of what food is supposed to do but can't
without the named nutrients. That is to nourish
and cleanse the body. The repercussions of long
term consumption of such foods are
constipation and an accumulation of toxins for

132

which the body builds up fat or tumors as
storage spaces, as well as chronic diseases of the
digestive tract and related organs, allergies,
musculoskeletal- and cardiovascular problems,
and autoimmune diseases (incl. AIDS).

Nutrition and Brain Function
http://www.ars.usda.gov/is/AR/archive/aug07/aging080
7.htm

Top 100 High ORAC Value Antioxidant Foods
http://modernsurvivalblog.com/health/high-orac-value-
antioxidant-foods-top-100/

Early dementia often caused by autoimmune disorders
http://www.reuters.com/article/2008/04/15/us-early-
dementia-often-caused-autoimmun-
idUSPAT57989320080415

Autoimmune Causes of Dementia
http://elaine-moore.suite101.com/autoimmune-causes-
of-dementia-a293654

Causes Of Early Onset Dementia
http://www.livestrong.com/article/118117-causes-early-
onset-dementia/

How To Eat To Lose Weight
http://www.heavenministries.com/health/how_to_eat_to_
lose_weight_copyri.htm

Soil Temperature
http://www.essortment.com/soil-temperature-54558.html

Review: Maximize Immunity (Comby)
http://www.beyondveg.com/nieft-k/rvw/rvw-maximize-
immunity.shtml

Denaturation Protein
http://www.elmhurst.edu/~chm/vchembook/568denatur
ation.html

**How Can Constipation Function as a Root Cause of All
Disease and Illness?**
http://www.healthbeginsinthecolon.com/chapter-
summaries.html

133

"Sometimes I think my head is so big because it is so full of dreams," He might have been speaking for the Boskops, an almost forgotten group of early humans who lived in southern Africa between 30,000-10,000 years ago. The Boskops were similar to modern humans but had small, childlike faces and huge melon heads that held brains about 30% larger than our own.

The Extinct Human Species That Was Smarter Than Us
http://discovermagazine.com/2008/mar/21-the-extinct-human-species-that-was-smarter-than-us

Factory

Industrial agriculture also creates hunger and malnutrition at another level – by robbing crops of nutrients. Industrially produced food is a nutritionally 'empty mass', loaded with chemicals and toxins. Nutrition in food comes from the nutrients in the soil. Industrial agriculture, based on synthetic nitrogen –, phosphorus –, and potassium – based fertilisers, leads to the depletion of vital micronutrients and trace elements such as magnesium, zinc, calcium and iron.

Swaraj: A Deeper Freedom
http://www.vandanashiva.org/?p=611

Modern industrial agriculture is operated by a small number of corporations and consists of Concentrated (or Confined) Animal Feeding Operations (CAFOs) and monocultural crop fields, biotech laboratories, agrochemical- and food factories; local-, state-, and international trade, and public relations, advertising, wholesale, and retail.

Agribusiness animals exist in conditions that are unsanitary and further deteriorate the quality of the resulting food. They are fed a mush consisting of genetically engineered grains, pharmaceuticals and other chemicals, plastic pellets (artificial roughage), rendered animal carcasses, manure/litter, blood, feathers, hairs and skins.

Agribusiness plant foods are doused with pesticides, herbicides, fungicides, heavy metals, CAFO manure/litter, and artificial fertilizers. Increasingly, fruits (incl. sugar cane), vegetables, fish, cattle, sheep, and goats are being genetically engineered and/or otherwise manipulated to reach specific criteria, most of which focus on short term profits rather than the quality of the product.

The quality of a food product is measured by its taste, aroma, and texture, all of which reflect its nutritional density. The nutritional density of a food product is dependent on the health of the soil, the water, the air, and the plant itself. In the case of animals, the nutritional quality of animal products depends on all of the above, as well as on the treatment of the animal by humans. To achieve superior food quality, farmers must be small scale, private, organic, and operating in ways that are as close to natural as possible, while accepting the fact that

135

certain plants, animals, and sea creatures cannot be domesticated.

Ultimately, even if people lived in an environment that was completely free of industrial pollution, stress, and worry, industrial food alone would literally destroy their gastrointestinal function.

The Issues: Factory Farming
http://www.sustainabletable.org/issues/factoryfarming/

Factory Farms
http://www.foodandwaterwatch.org/food/factoryfarms/

Living a Nightmare: Animal Factories in Michigan
http://video.google.com/videoplay?docid=5163144866474931803

IS YOUR MEAT FIT TO EAT IS YOUR MEAT FIT TO EAT
beyondfactoryfarming.org/files/BFF_Brochure07.pdf

How sustainable agriculture can address the environmental and human health harms of industrial agriculture
http://www.ncbi.nlm.nih.gov/pmc/articles/PMC1240832/

The Meatrix
http://www.themeatrix.com/

Agrochemical
http://en.wikipedia.org/wiki/Agrochemical

Agriculture
http://en.wikipedia.org/wiki/Agriculture

Industrial agriculture (crops)
http://en.wikipedia.org/wiki/Industrial_agriculture_(crops)

Monoculture
http://en.wikipedia.org/wiki/Monoculture

They Eat What? The Reality of Feed at Animal Factories
http://www.ucsusa.org/food_and_agriculture/science_an
d_impacts/impacts_industrial_agriculture/they-eat-what-
the-reality-of.html
Genetically modified food
http://en.wikipedia.org/wiki/Genetically_modified_food
GMO Fruit Facts
http://www.youtube.com/watch?v=-qCS19sK6h0
Talking Fruit: How To Tell If Fruit Is Genetically Modified
http://www.plantea.com/genetically-modified-foods.htm
Seven Deadly Myths of Industrial Agriculture
http://www.ehow.com/about_5195502_seven-deadly-
myths-industrial-agriculture.html
Why Agriculture?
http://nashvilleurbanharvest.org/pages/why-get-
involved-in-agriculture
Exploring the Link Between Animal Health and Food Safety
http://www.foodsafetynews.com/2012/05/exploring-the-
link-between-animal-health-and-food-safety/
Raj Patel Discusses Stuffed & Starved
http://rajpatel.org/2009/11/11/raj-patel-discusses-
stuffed-starved/
Genetic Chile
http://vimeo.com/11416802
How can you keep kosher when your rice pudding has human DNA in it?
http://www.opednews.com/articles/GMOs-and-JEWS---
Muslims-by-Linn-Cohen-Cole-090211-386.html
FRESH the movie
http://www.freshthemovie.com/

When we examine how our food is grown today, it becomes clear that most of the chemical tools taken for granted by modern agribusiness are products of

warfare. Is this merely an indirect consequence of the tragic history of the 20th century, or does it suggest that the currently dismal state of our soils, fresh water supplies and rural economies is an outgrowth of agribusiness emergence from wartime in some important ways? Virtually all of the leading companies that brought us chemical fertilizers and pesticides made their greatest fortunes during wartime. How can this help us understand the ever-deteriorating quality of mass produced food?
Agribusiness, Biotechnology and War
http://www.social-ecology.org/2002/09/agribusiness-biotechnology-and-war/

"So Long Constipation, Part 1" is available in paperback, ebook, and audiobook format on Amazon, Google Play, Smashwords, iTunes, Audible, and Barnes and Noble.